# FATIGUE and
# DYSAUTONOMIA

# CHRONIC FATIGUE SYNDROME

### also known as

# MYALGIC ENCEPHALOMYELITIS

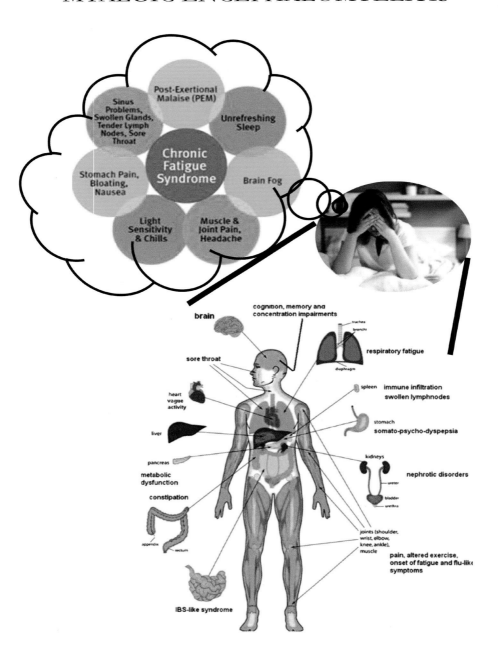

# FATIGUE AND DYSAUTONOMIA

## Chronic or Persistent, What's the Difference?

### The Mind-Body Wellness Program

(adapted from *Clinical Autonomic and Mitochondrial Disorders— Diagnosis, Prevention, and Treatment for Mind-Body Wellness*)

by
### Nicholas L. DePace, MD, FACC
and
### Joseph Colombo, PhD, DNM, DHS

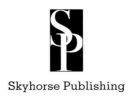

Skyhorse Publishing

Skyhorse Publishing books may be purchased in bulk at special discounts for sales promotion, corporate gifts, fund-raising, or educational purposes. Special editions can also be created to spec- ifications. For details, contact the Special Sales Department, Skyhorse Publishing, 307 West 36th Street, 11th Floor, New York, NY 10018 or info@skyhorsepublishing.com.

Skyhorse® and Skyhorse Publishing® are registered trademarks of Skyhorse Publishing, Inc.®, a Delaware corporation.

Visit our website at www.skyhorsepublishing.com.

10 9 8 7 6 5 4 3 2 1

Library of Congress Cataloging-in-Publication Data is available on file.

Print ISBN: 978-1-5107-6089-9
eBook ISBN: 978-1-5107-6117-9

Cover design by Kai Texel

Printed in China

# CONTENTS

# ABBREVIATIONS

| | |
|---|---|
| AAD | Advanced Autonomic Dysfunction (similar to DAN, without the diabetes) |
| AFib | Atrial Fibrillation |
| ALA | Alpha-Lipoic Acid |
| ANS | Autonomic Nervous System |
| ATP | Adenosine Triphosphate |
| BP | Blood Pressure |
| CAN | Cardiovascular Autonomic Neuropathy |
| CFS | Chronic Fatigue Syndrome |
| CoQ10 | Coenzyme Q10 |
| DAN | Diabetic Autonomic Neuropathy (similar to AAD, with diabetes) |
| EDS | Ehlers-Danlos Syndrome |
| FDA | United States Food and Drug Administration |
| GI | Gastrointestinal |
| HR | Heart Rate |
| LFa | Low Frequency area, the Sympathetic measure |
| ME | Myalgic Encephalomyelitis |
| OD | Orthostatic Dysfunction |
| OI | Orthostatic Intolerance |
| P&S | Parasympathetic and Sympathetic |
| PE | a "dynamic" Parasympathetic Excess |
| PEM | Post-Exertional Malaise |
| POTS | Postural Orthostatic Tachycardia Syndrome |
| PTSD | Post-Traumatic Stress Disorder |
| QoL | Quality of Life |
| RFa | Respiratory Frequency area, the Parasympathetic measure |
| SB | Sympathovagal Balance (=[resting LFa]/[resting RFa]) |
| SE | Sympathetic Excess |
| SW | Sympathetic Withdrawal |
| VTach | Ventricular Tachycardia |

# CONTENT FORMAT

After the Introduction (including the Background, Mind-Body Wellness Program Basics, Parasympathetic and Sympathetic (P&S) monitoring, and Disclaimers), the main body of the book is written in two parts (see the next spread as the example): one part to the patient or the patient's loved ones and one part to the physicians. The patient part is written on the right-hand page (the odd-numbered pages) and the physician part is written on the left-hand page (the even-numbered pages). Essentially the same information is presented in both parts, just using different styles ("languages") to communicate the information. In this way, patients (if interested) may see what the doctors may be, or as we believe should be, considering, and the physicians will have an example of a way of communicating with their patients, especially in the autonomic field which is poorly understood and even less well taught.

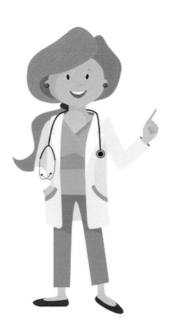

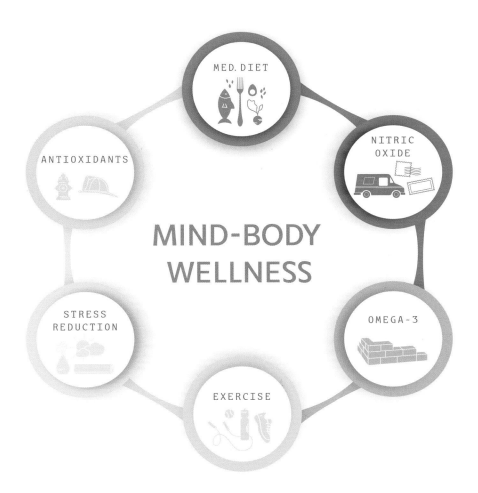

# FOR PHYSICIANS

*In the main body of the book, left-hand (or even-numbered) pages are written for physicians.*

While other Dysautonomia books explain how to manage patients with autonomic dysfunction, we look to provide more information to help physicians treat autonomic dysfunction (aka Dysautonomia). Furthermore, assuming no end-organ damage or genetic causes, we believe the recommendations herein will help physicians to work with their patients to restore health and even wellness, if certain lifestyles are adopted.

This book will lean heavily toward supplements and lifestyle treatments for fatigue and Dysautonomia. The primary reason is that there are only two pharmaceuticals (Midodrine and Northera) approved for autonomic dysfunction. All other pharmaceuticals that are recommended are off-label recommendations. In fact, there are now more supplements and lifestyles recommended in large, multicenter studies for dysautonomia (including dosing; e.g., alpha-lipoic acid, fish oil, coenzyme Q10, and exercise) than approved pharmaceuticals.

We include information to enable the physician to provide:

- Thorough, clinical assessments,
- Patient education upon diagnosis,
- Assistance with interpreting and understanding the results of Parasympathetic and Sympathetic (P&S) monitoring,
- Possible therapy options, including short-term, long-term, and lifelong.

*Continued on page 4 . . .*

# FOR PATIENTS AND THEIR LOVED ONES

*In the main body of the book, right hand (or odd-numbered) pages are written for patients.*

While other Dysautonomia books explain how you the patient should live with autonomic dysfunction (aka Dysautonomia), we look to help you to overcome your Dysautonomia and associated fatigue. As we have helped countless numbers of patients in the past, we hope to help you to reclaim your life by improving your quality of life and reducing the numbers of symptoms, medications, and costs associated with fatigue.

As we have, and continue to do, these general therapy recommendations must be tailored specifically to you the individual patient. Therefore, the recommendations herein are not "one size fits all." They must be considered by your physician specifically for you in light of your individual medical and personal history. Please do not consider any statement in this book as a diagnosis or prescribed therapy plan. These are guidelines to help educate. Again, THE INFORMATION IN THIS BOOK MUST BE CONSIDERED BY A PHYSICIAN AND APPLIED BY A PHYSICIAN BASED ON YOUR CLINICAL HISTORY.

We hope that the information contained herein will restore hope for a better life and faith in the healthcare system, to enable you to work with your physician toward wellness. While not everyone, we have indeed helped most patients become active again and return to being a contributor to society. This is not to say that you may not need therapy lifelong. In fact, most do. However, the therapy may not require pharmaceuticals.

*Continued on page 5 . . .*

THE INFORMATION IN THIS BOOK IS NOT **FDA** APPROVED. IT IS MEANT ONLY AS RECOMMENDATIONS FOR YOUR CONSIDERATION, GIVEN THE MEDICAL AND INDIVIDUAL HISTORY AND CURRENT CONDITION OF YOUR INDIVIDUAL PATIENT. PLEASE DO NOT CONSIDER ANY STATEMENT IN THIS BOOK AS A DIAGNOSIS OR PRESCRIBED THERAPY PLAN. THESE ARE GUIDELINES TO HELP EDUCATE.

The primary basis for this book is the science text: DePace NL and Colombo J. *Clinical Autonomic and Mitochondrial Disorders—Diagnosis, Prevention, and Treatment for Mind-Body Wellness.* Springer Science + Business Media, New York, NY, 2019 [1]. For a more in-depth discussion on P&S monitoring consider the science text: Colombo J, Arora RR, DePace NL, Vinik AI. *Clinical Autonomic Dysfunction: Measurement, Indications, Therapies, and Outcomes.* Springer Science + Business Media, New York, NY, 2014 [2]. This book focuses the science on fatigue in a less formal style. Enjoy!

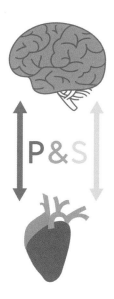

We include information to educate you the patient so that you may work better with your physician and achieve health and wellness. To this end, we explain:

- How the P&S branches of the autonomic nervous system should work together, in balance;
- How Dysautonomia (P&S imbalance) contributes to your symptoms of fatigue;
- Why you may not have been properly diagnosed in the past;
- The clinical differences between Chronic and persistent fatigue;
- What to expect in working with your physician; and
- How to help.

Be Well!

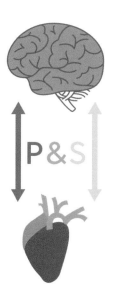

# INTRODUCTION

## Background

Fatigue: chronic or persistent? Chronic Fatigue Syndrome (CFS) is a specifically defined disorder (or syndrome). As such, not all patients that complain of fatigue fit the classification. As a result, not all patients that complain of fatigue are well treated, and some of those that do fit (or are force-fitted) into the CFS classification are perhaps overmedicated or ill-served. Those that do not fit, or should not fit the CFS classification, we will suggest that they have "persistent fatigue."

This still leaves the question: "How do we differentiate the two and thereby better define treatment?"

Measurements from the Autonomic Nervous System (ANS), specifically the Parasympathetic and Sympathetic (P&S) Nervous Systems is more information [2]. First, it is not only more information from a generalized population perspective. It is more information that is specific to the individual patient. From our experience, this more specific information, when added to the patient's own history and physiology, enables physicians to refine the classification and plan more individualized therapy and treatment. Treatment that is based on, and therefore more specific to, your (the patient's) own history and individual physiology.

## 17 MILLION PEOPLE AND GROWING

You are not alone! CFS (also known as Myalgic Encephalomyelitis, collectively referred to as ME/CFS) is estimated to affect over 17 million people worldwide, according to the ME Action Network, a world-wide advocacy group. In the United States alone, the CDC estimates that over 880,000 people are diagnosed with ME/CFS, but believes that over 2.5 million is the actual number. This suggests that 1.62 million are left undiagnosed. If this ratio is applied to the world-wide number, then there is an estimated 48.3 million people suffering from CFS with about 65 percent of them undiagnosed. This number does not include what we are calling persistent fatigue, which may accompany depression, anxiety, hypermobility (Ehlers-Danlos Syndrome, aka EDS, a collagen gene disease), heart disease, multiple sclerosis and many other neurological diseases, overmedication, and more. ME/CFS, specifically, is known to affect women more than men; approximately 75 percent of ME/CFS patients are female and 25 percent are male, and it is estimated that up to 90 percent are undiagnosed. Of those diagnosed, up to 75 percent are unable to work, up to 25 percent are housebound or bedridden, and only about 5 percent are known to recover. These are appalling statistics. More information is needed to improve these statistics.

You may have also heard CFS called Systemic Exertion Intolerance Disease. To prevent confusion we will stay with either CFS or persistent fatigue. Again, CFS has a very specific set of criteria upon which it is diagnosed, and is therefore differentiated from "persistent" fatigue. In our terminology, persistent fatigue applies to everyone else who is *persistently* fatigued and not diagnosed with CFS.

## CHARACTERISTICS

Symptoms of Myalgic Encephalomyelitis/Chronic Fatigue Syndrome (ME/CFS) may appear similar to many other illnesses, and there is no test to confirm ME/CFS. This makes ME/CFS difficult to diagnose. The illness can be unpredictable. Symptoms may come and go, or there may be changes in how bad they are over time.

To distinguish ME/CFS from other illnesses, a doctor will need to do a thorough medical exam. This includes asking many questions about the patient's health history (physical and mental) and current illness and medications and asking about the symptoms to learn how often they occur, how bad they are, and how long they have lasted, and may also include ordering a number of lab and clinical tests. It is also important for doctors to talk with patients about how the symptoms affect their lives.

CFS is a complex of symptoms characterized by fatigue for a long period of time, usually more than six months, in which a person's daily activities are significantly curtailed. As indicated above, a great majority of patients become disabled or are unable to maintain gainful employment. Also, quality of life (QoL) is severely affected. There are many definitions for the term "Chronic Fatigue Syndrome" or the alternates. These definitions have changed over time. Significant problems with post-exertional fatigue are a hallmark of this syndrome. Also, sleep problems, autonomic dysfunction with orthostatic-related symptoms, cognitive impairment, and memory impairments are part of the disorder.

Five primary symptoms that are required for diagnosis are:

- Greatly lowered ability to do activities that were usual before the illness. This drop in activity level occurs along with fatigue and must last six months or longer. People with ME/CFS have fatigue that is very different from just being tired. The fatigue of ME/CFS is not relieved by sleep or rest.
- Worsening of ME/CFS symptoms after physical or mental activity (including just taking a shower) that would not have caused a problem before illness. This is known as post-exertional malaise (PEM). People with ME/CFS often describe this experience as a "crash," "relapse," or "collapse." During PEM, any ME/CFS symptoms may get worse or first appear, including difficulty thinking, problems sleeping, sore throat, headaches, feeling dizzy, or severe tiredness. It may take days, weeks, or longer to recover from a crash. Sometimes patients may be housebound or even completely bedbound during crashes. People with ME/CFS may not be able to predict what

will cause a crash or how long it will last.

- Sleep problems. People with ME/CFS may not feel better or less tired, even after a full night of sleep. Some people with ME/CFS may have problems falling asleep or staying asleep.
- Problems with thinking and memory. Most people with ME/CFS have trouble thinking quickly, remembering things, and paying attention to details. Patients often say they have "brain fog" to describe this problem because they feel "stuck in a fog" and not able to think clearly.
- Pain is very common in people with ME/CFS, but not all have pain. The type of pain, where it occurs, and how bad it is varies a lot: muscle pain (including "coat hanger" pain, which is a pain between the shoulder blades and up the neck, and myalgias), joint pain (polyarthralgias), digestive pain (including sore throat), tender lymph nodes, new headaches, or other generalized pain syndromes. The pain patients with ME/CFS feel is not caused by an injury. These pain syndromes are also associated with EDS and postural orthostatic tachycardia syndrome (POTS), both of which involved dysautonomias.

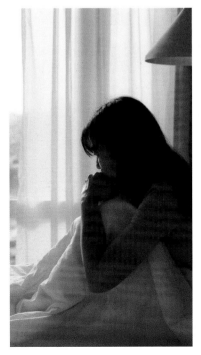

Another common complaint is worsening of symptoms while standing or sitting upright. This is called orthostatic intolerance. People with ME/CFS may be light-headed, dizzy, weak, or faint while standing or sitting up. They may have vision changes like blurring or seeing spots.

The cause of CFS is not known. Dysregulation of the Autonomic

**Introduction**

Nervous System has been implicated, as well as infection, immune system abnormalities, and mitochondrial dysfunction. However, CFS is correlated with Autonomic disease [3–7] and mitochondrial disease [8–10], and may be a result of both. Note: The autonomic and mitochondrial implications are the reasons for the writing of this book to focus our approach as published in the science text: DePace NL and Colombo J. *Clinical Autonomic and Mitochondrial Disorders—Diagnosis, Prevention, and Treatment for Mind-Body Wellness.* Springer Science + Business Media, New York, NY, 2019. An association with certain genetic markers or a history of childhood trauma may be causal factors. Studies on genetics have shown a familial predisposition of CFS, although the studies have been small. Because CFS may cause sore throat, lymphadenopathy, arthralgias, and muscle pain, it has been linked to the immune system and inflammatory process. Most of the studies have been inconclusive regarding characteristic immune features of CFS. Childhood trauma is implicated since CFS seems to affect children and teenagers more than adults, although fatigue is also common in adults over forty years of age. In general, the effects of trauma, including Post-Traumatic Stress Disorder (PTSD) and concussion, also involve fatigue.

ME/CFS is a heterogeneous group of patients. Recent studies [11–15] suggest triggering insults such as infections can cause autoantibodies and oxidative stress to dysregulate cellular and specifically mitochondrial energetics (see figures, next two pages), both of which may lead to exercise intolerance. Other common symptoms of ME/CFS may be due to (1) disturbed gut microbiota possibly leading to "leaky-gut" or other GI consequences; (2) microglial activation and inflammation of the nervous system, including the central nervous system, possibly leading to chronic pain due to allodynia and hyperalgesia; (3) neuronal inflammation is important in the pathophysiology of creating many disabling symptoms; (4) high levels of pro-inflammatory cytokines and low levels of antioxidants, such as CoQ10 or Glutathione,

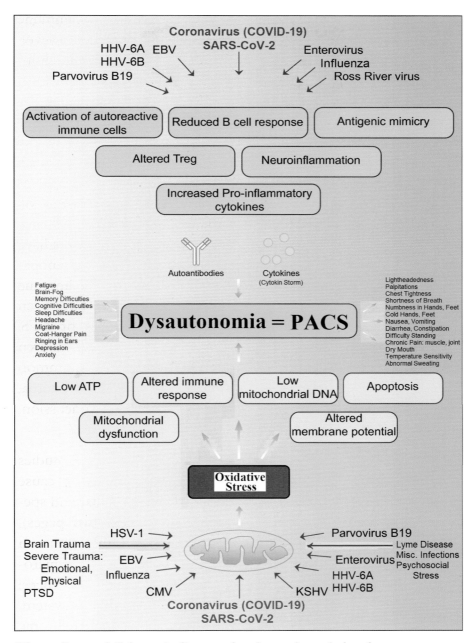

**Figure Legend**: Schematic diagram showing various viral pathogens potentially associated with ME/CFS and possible molecular mechanisms altered by these pathogens that can contribute to ME/CFS development [adapted from 16].

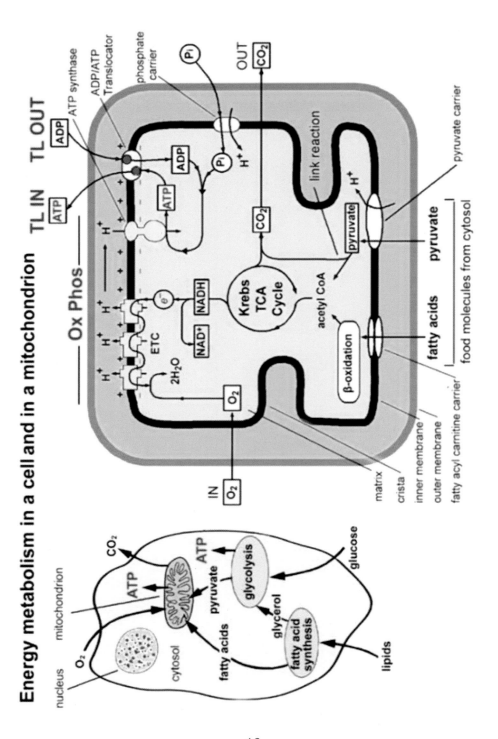

Energy metabolism in a cell and in a mitochondrion

**Figure Legend (opposite page):** Main stages and location of energy metabolism in a human cell (left), and simplified details of a mitochondrion showing the main metabolic cycles and the oxidative phosphorylation respiratory chain (right). The outer mitochondrial membrane is highly permeable whereas the inner membrane is permeable only to water and gases. Special carrier and Translocator proteins pass reactants through it. At the top are the proteins involved in the respiratory electron transfer chain (ETC) and in the transfer of ATP and ADP between the cytosol and mitochondrion. ADP and $P_i$ are combined by ATP synthase to make ATP. The ADP/ATP Translocator opens OUT to transfer ADP into the matrix and opens IN to transfer ATP to the cytosol. Nicotinamide adenine dinucleotide plays a key role in its oxidized form $NAD^+$ and its reduced form $NADH + H^+$ in carrying and transferring protons ($H^+$) and electrons ($e^-$) [17].

have been reported; or (5) abnormalities of the Hypothalamus-Pituitary-Adrenal Axis possibly leading to "delayed cortisol awakening" possibly leading to unrefreshing sleep. We recommend ALA because Glutathione does not penetrate into the mitochondria whereas ALA does and helps to recycle Glutathione, along with many other benefits.

Researchers [17] used an Adenosine Triphosphate (ATP) profile test (see Appendix 1) in neutrophils to establish mitochondrial dysfunction in ME/CSF patients. They concluded "our observations strongly implicate mitochondrial dysfunction as the *immediate* cause of CFS symptoms (see figures, previous three pages). However, we cannot tell whether the damage to mitochondrial function is a primary effect or secondary effect to one or more of a number of comorbidities, for example, cellular hypoxia or oxidative stress, including excessive peroxynitrates." A familial aggregation of ME/CFS has been noted. Metabolic differences in ME/CFS patients demonstrate inability of CFS Peripheral Blood Mononuclear Cells (PBMCS) to fulfill cellular energetic demands both under basal conditions and when mitochondria are stressed during periods of high metabolic demand such as hypoglycemia.

The concurrence of similar autoantibodies in patients with POTS [17] (which may be comorbid with vasovagal syncope) and ME/CFS (particularly muscarinic and adrenergic receptor abnormalities) is more than coincidental. Parasympathetic and Sympathetic dysfunction and ME/CFS are apparently "joined at the hip." Ehlers-Danlos Syndrome (EDS) and hypermobile patients may have a genetic predisposition to autoimmunity and mitochondrial dysfunction. Many of these patients also manifest autonomic (P&S) dysfunction and ME/CFS. POTS, EDS and ME/CFS all have significant fatigue as a common symptom with a "dynamic" Parasympathetic Excess (PE) as a common dysautonomia. PE is central to vasovagal syncope [18]. Many of the symptoms of EDS or hypermobility are due to "leaky" connective tissue which causes an excessively active immune system, which is associated with PE since the Parasympathetics control the immune system. We also find that PE is significantly associated with ME/CFS [18]. The adrenergic abnormalities may be explained by PE, including excessive adrenergic or Sympathetic activity. With PE, Sympathetic Excess is secondary, due to the Sympathetic response being abnormally amplified by the Parasympathetic increase (rather than the decrease that is expected to happen normally) [18]. In fact, we believe the autoimmunity to also be associated with PE. PE causes an overactive immune system, which in more normal patients may lead to autoimmunity. PE-mediated autoimmunity results from the immune system being excessively active, and having exhausted any invading entities, turns on the host. We have seen that relieving PE has relieved some autoimmune symptoms, especially in the absence of autoantibodies relating to that symptom [personal observation. A fully referenced and illustrated version of this previous section is available at https://franklincardiovascular.com].

CFS is classified by the World Health Organization as a chronic neurological condition [19]. CFS symptoms including palpitations, bowel and bladder dysfunction, dizziness, and temperature dysregulation are commonly seen and are regulated by the P&S nervous systems. This strongly suggests that P&S nervous system dysfunction (also known as Dysautonomia) is key in CFS. In fact, there is overlap between orthostatic intolerance (a cause of light-headedness upon standing and may involve significant fatigue) and decreases in postural blood pressure (postural hypotension) and multiple sclerosis and CFS [20]. The strongest relationship between CFS and the P&S nervous systems is shown between the association of CFS and postural orthostatic tachycardia syndrome (POTS). In POTS, the heart rate responses are abnormally high when standing, causing the patient to feel like they are running a marathon while standing still. A similar cause of mechanism with POTS and CFS has been postulated by many investigators [21,22]. However, P&S monitoring often finds challenge Parasympathetic Excess [23] (a type of Dysautonomia) more often than POTS; both produce similar symptoms. The Hypothalamic-Pituitary Axis (a major hormonal system within the body) has also been implicated in the cause of CFS with dysregulation of this axis being seen in many patients. Reduced cortisol levels and decreased variability of the Hypothalamic-Pituitary Axis have been found [24,25], but some of these results have also been inconsistent [26,27].

## INFLAMMATION IMPLICIT

Inflammation has been implicated. Inflammation is one of many Sympathetic functions. Cytokines and proteins have been shown to be abnormal in CFS, including various interleukins and tumor necrosis factors. However, again, studies have been inconsistent in these findings. The role of the immune system has been conflicting. Prognoses of CFS have had variable numbers. Studies point to patterns of recovery: 0-20 percent a full recovery, 8-63 percent some improvement in symptoms, 5-20 percent have worsening symptoms, 24-57 percent report no change [28]. The P&S nervous systems are invariably affected in this disorder. As a result of P&S dysfunction (Dysautonomia), baroreceptor reflex may be impaired. Baroreceptor reflex, a reflex controlled by the Sympathetic nervous system, ultimately controls blood pressure (BP). The wrong BP at the wrong time may cause fatigue. Many studies show a relationship between CFS and ANS dysfunction. The findings are not always reproducible, however. This may be due to the fact that only the ANS is being measured and not its two branches, the P&S nervous systems. As we will discuss later, ANS (as opposed to P&S) measures are measures of the sum total of the two P&S branches. As a result, ANS measures force assumption and approximation, most of which apply only to healthy individuals. A cross-sectional study using the COMPASS questionnaire showed that almost 90 percent of CFS patients experienced symptoms related to Dysautonomia from P&S dysfunction [29]. Overall, cost and expenditure of money has been very significant (including an annual cost of lost productivity in excess of $24 billion in the United States alone), and it seems to only be getting worse.

Chronic fatigue syndrome is characterized by debilitating fatigue that is not relieved with rest and is associated with physical symptoms. The Centers for Disease Control and Prevention criteria for chronic fatigue syndrome include severe fatigue lasting longer than six months, as well as presence of at least four of the following physical symptoms: post-exertional malaise; unrefreshing sleep; impaired memory or concentration; muscle pain; polyarthralgia; sore throat; tender lymph nodes; or new headaches. It is a clinical diagnosis that can be made only when other disease processes are excluded. [30]

As you can see, there is still much confusion in and around CFS. As a result, there is much controversy regarding appropriate therapies and treatment plans. Most attempt to treat the symptoms, or simply ignore it by referring to psychiatry. . . . Little wonder the vast majority are misdiagnosed, and even fewer find relief. More recently, with the legalization of marijuana, and the (largely unsubstantiated) claims of helping relieve fatigue, we see too much potential for this situation to only become worse, and significantly so.

Given that the P&S nervous systems control and coordinate all of the systems that underlie the symptoms of fatigue regardless of the cause, and the fact that mitochondria fuel all the needs of these systems, it may be that the more information from P&S monitoring will help to improve our understanding of ME/CFS and its corollary persistent fatigue.

With P&S monitoring, also known as Cardio-Respiratory Testing, abnormalities in P&S function are documented and medications are adjusted in an attempt to get better autonomic balance, both at rest, and dynamically (e.g., anticholinergic or sympatholytic therapy with Midodrine). Once the P&S systems are in balance, first dynamically, then at rest, many symptoms tend to be relieved. Symptoms that remain are the results of end-organ dysfunction and must be targeted to maintain P&S balance and health. In this way, P&S monitoring and P&S-guided therapy may help to resolve the confusion and controversy around fatigue, which seems to be a highly individualistic condition.

## SIX PRONGS

The six-prong supplement and lifestyle routine is recommended to reduce oxidative stress, including (1) antioxidants such as alpha-lipoic acid, CoQ10, L-carnitine, and vitamins to ensure mitochondrial health to provide more energy, (2) omega-3 fatty acids to reduce inflammation and help repair P&S nerve damage, (3) nitric oxide to ensure abundant blood flow and cardiovascular health, (4) exercise as the most powerful of antioxidants, (5) Mediterranean Diet to provide fuel and additional antioxidants and nitric oxide, and (6) psychosocial (whole-body) stress reduction, which is also an antioxidant. All six prongs address areas of research that have been shown to help relieve the symptoms of CFS, including by preserving mitochondrial health, helping to produce more energy at the cellular level as well as for the whole body. This then helps to restore P&S balance, which helps to relieve sleep and GI difficulties, reduce pain syndromes, and restore proper circulation (blood flow), especially to the brain to relieve memory and cognitive difficulties and relieve light-headedness and dizziness, and headache or migraine). Collectively, all of this helps to relieve fatigue.

# Mind-Body Wellness Program Basics

The brain and the heart are key to WELLNESS. They are connected to each other, and the rest of the body, by the Parasympathetic and Sympathetic (P&S) nervous systems and blood (via the vasculature). These systems control and coordinate all the other systems. Keeping these systems healthy and WELL helps to maintain WELLNESS throughout the rest of the systems of the body, and thereby MAXIMIZES QUALITY OF LIFE (by minimizing morbidity risk) and MAXIMIZES LONGEVITY (by minimizing mortality risk).

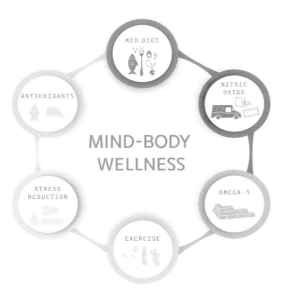

QUALITY OF LIFE, as defined for an adult, would include:

- eating and sleeping well,
- regular bathroom habits,
- having sex,
- normal blood pressure, and
- not getting dizzy or fatigued frequently.

The Mind-Body Wellness Program is designed to provide you MAXIMUM QUALITY OF LIFE and LONGEVITY. It does so by recommending its "Six prongs to WELLNESS:"

1. **Omega-3 Fatty Acids** is the membrane molecule. It provides the building blocks for our membranes, like the stones in a stone wall (as in the insert, right). However, unlike stones, omega-3 fatty acids also help to keep cell walls supple and receptive (represented by the flowers) to passing in to the cell the raw materials necessary to support WELLNESS, as well as passing out those which do not.

2. **Nitric Oxide** is the anti-atherosclerotic molecule. With a supporting cast of **amino acids, vitamins, and minerals**, it keeps the body operating as a WELL oiled machine. It is a policeman, regulating blood flow and preventing traffic jams (clots). It is a fireman, preventing inFLAMmation that causes white blood cells to adhere to blood vessel walls. It is a paramedic, repairing membranes throughout the body. It is an engineer, building new blood vessels (roads) to efficiently supply the entire body. It is also an antioxidant.

3. **Antioxidants** (**alpha-lipoic acid** and **CoQ10**) to prevent stress at the cellular level from both inflammation and oxidative stress (oxidation is burning—a fire is an oxidation reaction). They keep the immune system and the power plants of the body—the **mitochondria**–WELL. In fact, antioxidants support the health of all systems throughout the body, and help to keep them healthy, energized, and WELL.

The three lifestyle prongs (following) of the **Mind-Body Wellness Program** all provide antioxidant protection. In fact, exercise may just be the most potent of all antioxidant processes. These two particular antioxidants (alpha-lipoic acid and CoQ10) are the most powerful, natural antioxidants we have. Your body produces them. Not only are they the most powerful in and of themselves, they make themselves even more powerful by recycling other antioxidants, like vitamins A, C, and E. Without alpha-lipoic acid (ALA) and CoQ10, these vitamins typically make only one pass through the body. Note, the reason why the literature has so many differing opinions on the efficacy and dosing of these vitamins as antioxidants is because most experiments (assuming they were actually performed) did not account for the level of ALA or CoQ10. ALA and CoQ10 are both produced in the human body, and that production decreases with age and duration of chronic disease.

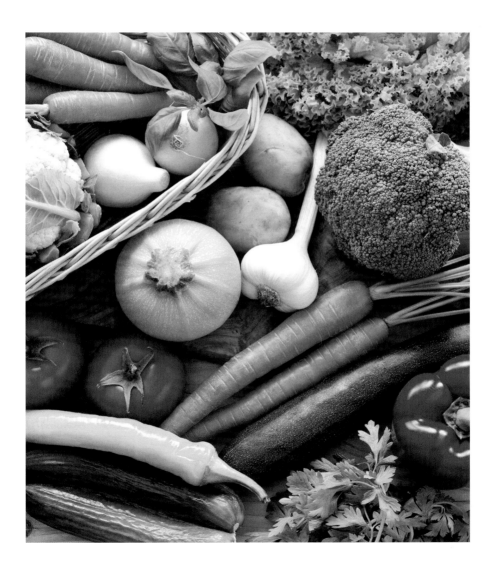

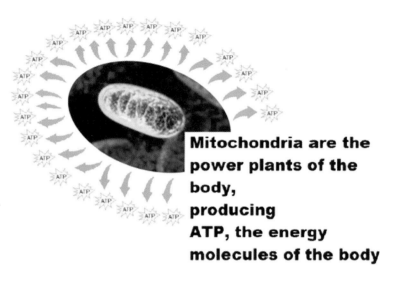

**Mitochondria are the power plants of the body, producing ATP, the energy molecules of the body**

4. <u>**Mediterranean Diet**</u> is a lifestyle to fuel our bodies with the ingredients required for WELLNESS, while avoiding ingredients that promote the diseases of our time that are becoming epidemic (over fifteen types of cancer, dementia, atherosclerosis, and diabetes). It includes eating mostly whole grains, fruits, and vegetables. The protein is obtained from eating mostly fish and seafood, lean meats, eggs, cheese, yogurt, and milk. It includes very few processed fats and sugars. The lifestyle aspect is that it mostly includes fresh, in-season, unprocessed foods: "factory fresh" (as in fresh from nature) not "fresh from the factory." The other lifestyle aspect is the way food is consumed. It should be consumed in a relaxed environment, at a table, with friends and family laughing and talking together. All of this good food and good company may be aided by a small glass of wine.

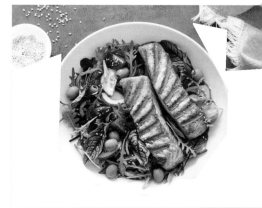

5. **Exercise**. *It is not a dirty word!* It is a fountain of youth lifestyle for WELLNESS. Think of it in terms of an active lifestyle. The lifestyle that preceded automobiles, elevators, television remotes, and cell phones. Examples include common housework, gardening, walking, and taking the stairs. It does not have to include going to the gym or beating yourself up to feel good. In fact, if you only feel good while exercising and feel more pain and fatigue after exercise, you may be exercising too hard, and your body may be perceiving that level of exercise as a stress, albeit a healthy stress. We are not discouraging those who do work out harder, and benefit from it and enjoy it, but it is not the minimum requirement. The recommended minimum is 150 minutes of moderate exercise per week. Perhaps a little more for young children.

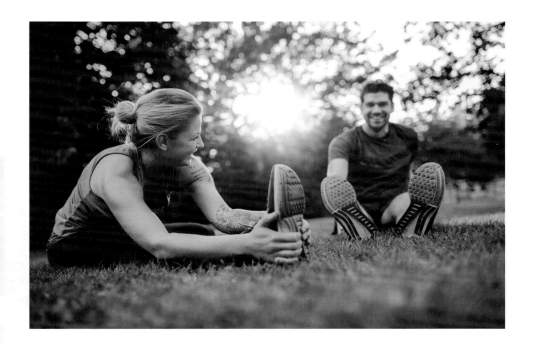

6. **<u>Psychosocial Stress Reduction</u>** is a lifestyle to prevent stress at the system level, promoting a happy, *"laughter is the best medicine,"* kind of WELLNESS.

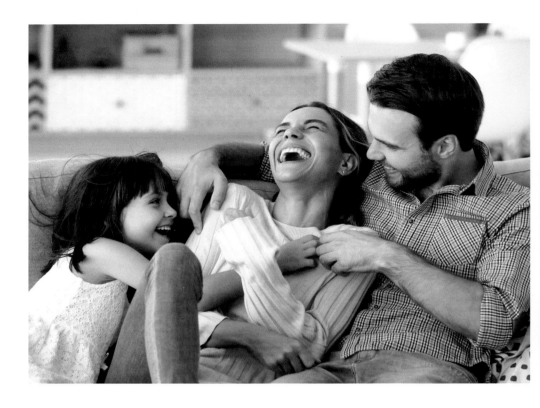

*The Mediterranean Diet and exercise work together to provide the foundations for health and WELLNESS. Exercise and psychosocial stress reduction help to keep the body happy, reduce pain and inflammation, enabling you to enjoy your health and WELLNESS!*

*All SIX PRONGS are important, and
are to be taken together as a whole!*

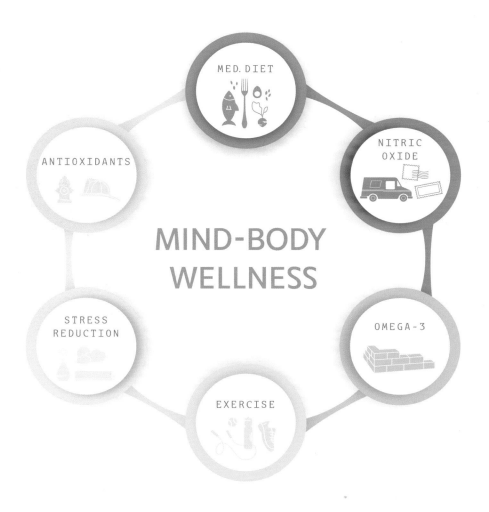

# Parasympathetic and Sympathetic Monitoring

Parasympathetic and Sympathetic (P&S) monitoring provides more information, helping to improve differential diagnoses and therapy planning. This more information may also help to identify disease and disorder earlier, even before symptoms present. P&S monitoring goes beyond customized medicine, promoting "individualized" medicine. As a result, it may reduce medication load, hospitalization and re-hospitalization, reduce morbidity and mortality risk, improve patient outcomes, and thereby reduce healthcare costs. Morbidity risks directly affect quality of life, and Mortality risks directly affect length of life. Establishing and maintaining P&S balance goes a long way toward BEING WELL.

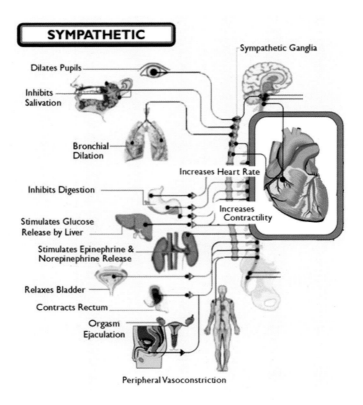

The P&S nervous system's responses collectively constitute an individual patient's physiologic "fingerprint." It may provide more information to help to reduce medication load (assuming no end-organ effects) by providing more information about the underlying disease state or disorder. A typical chronic disease patient, whose symptoms are being treated one at a time, may be prescribed three agents for high blood pressure, two medications for GI symptoms, two medications for sleep disorder, and one or more medications for anxiety; and may still have a poor quality of life. All of these symptoms (perhaps due to Anxiety, for example) may be due to Parasympathetic dysfunction (with any Sympathetic abnormalities secondary to the Parasympathetic dysfunction), which may be treated with one medication and a low-dose medication at that.

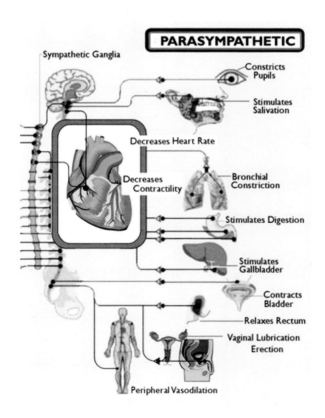

Relieving Parasympathetic dysfunction may relieve all of the others, including (eventually) the Sympathetic dysfunction and its related symptoms. Once Parasympathetic dysfunction is relieved, the patient may not need to stay on the medication (again, assuming no end-organ effects), for the nervous system learns and by this method may be "retrained" to maintain a new and healthier balance.

Continuing the Anxiety example, many Anxiety patients believe they are having a heart attack and visit the emergency room (ER). After testing, many patients still refuse to believe they are not having a heart attack and will not leave the ER. These patients continue to feel shortness of breath, chest tightness, and palpitations. However, if these symptoms are demonstrated to not be from a heart attack, then they are often a result of the "adrenaline storm" produced by the brain to call for more oxygenated blood. The shortness of breath is to make you breathe more to increase blood oxygenation. The chest tightness and palpitations are the body's responses to the increase in adrenaline that is spurring on the increase in blood pressure and heart rate (respectively) to increase blood flow to the brain. Not only does this consume resources unnecessarily, but it also includes unnecessary transportation costs. Remote P&S monitoring avoids all of these costs, helping to keep the patient at home.

To review, the Parasympathetic and Sympathetic branches of the autonomic nervous system work synergistically to control and coordinate the function of all bodily systems and virtually every cell in the body. The Sympathetics are the "fight or flight" system. They are the reactionary system. Sympathetic responses are meant to be short in duration (relative to the Parasympathetics), working in the acute phase of systemic responses to stresses (whether healthy or not). They react to the physiologic, or metabolic, threshold set by the Parasympathetics. To develop a useful analogy, they are like the accelerator of a car. In many instances, they accelerate functions of the body. Yet they are the slower of the two branches to respond. As in a car, you never want the accelerator working faster than the brakes, or you may not be able to stop the car and may crash. In the body, examples of the "crash" are a heart attack or a stroke. The majority of the Sympathetic nervous system outside the brain arises from the Sympathetic Chain ganglia just outside the spine (see previous two figures). There are other components to it as well, including the Angiotensin-Renin-Aldosterone system. Of course, the adrenal glands, including adrenaline and cortisol, are significant factors that influence and are influenced by the Sympathetics. The Sympathetics uniquely control the vasculature. The most common manifestations of Sympathetic responses are changes in HR & BP, as well as histaminergic and other inflammatory responses.

The Parasympathetics are the "rest and digest" system. As mentioned, they set the metabolic and physiologic thresholds around which the Sympathetics react, in any given situation. Parasympathetic responses are meant to be more chronic, although protracted Parasympathetic responses are also unhealthy, as in brain injury (concussion or trauma) or some conditions thought to be autoimmune. They are the protective branch of the autonomic nervous system, ensuring proper tissue perfusion throughout the body (that is why long Valsalva maneuvers are very strong Parasympathetic stimuli, short Valsalva maneuvers are powerful Sympathetic stimuli). When the body has been insulted too often or too traumatically, the Parasympathetics may remain activated for too long, causing many diffuse, seemingly unrelated, symptoms and causing the patient to be difficult to manage, especially regarding BP, blood sugars, hormones, and weight. The majority of the Parasympathetic nervous system outside the brain is the Vagus Nerve (see figure above). Of course, there are also Sacral, Nitrergic, and Enteric nerves that also carry Parasympathetic information. The Parasympathetics uniquely control the GI tract, outside the Enteric Nervous System (although the Enteric system is considered by most to be part of the Parasympathetic nervous system). The most common manifestations of P&S responses are Respiratory Sinus Arrhythmia (a Parasympathetic reflex during breathing) and gastric motility ("butterflies in the stomach" in response to stress, a Sympathetic response).

P&S balance directly affects morbidity and mortality risks, including quality of life. Adult quality of life may be defined as eating and sleeping well, proper bowel and bladder function, proper sex function, and normal BP and orthostatic responses. All of these are controlled or coordinated by the P&S nervous systems.

Again, the P&S nervous systems are like the brakes and accelerator of the body, respectively. Under normal conditions, for common activities, the following analogy describes the interaction between the P&S systems. As in a car (with an automatic transmission), if you are at a red light with your foot on the brakes and the light turns green, what is the first thing you do? . . . You take your foot off the brakes. Even before you touch the accelerator, you begin to roll, you already begin to accelerate. Taking your foot off the brakes minimizes the amount gas (read that as adrenaline) and acceleration (read that as Sympathetic stress) you need to reach your desired speed. The P&S nervous systems normally act in much the same manner: first the Parasympathetics decrease to facilitate and minimize the Sympathetic response, and then the Sympathetics increase.

Note, this does not exclude the "seesaw" model of the ANS taught in medical school. According to the "seesaw" model, normally when one branch is active (high), the other branch is not active (low). However, this occurs mostly in healthy subjects, and rarely in patients. The "seesaw" model is inherent in the "brake and accelerator" model. Normally, when one's foot is on the gas, there is not a foot on the brakes, and vice versa. The benefit of the "brake and accelerator" model is that is goes further in explaining many abnormal conditions. For example, Parasympathetic Excess with Sympathetic Excess (the autonomic dysfunction associated with Depression-Anxiety syndromes). In the "seesaw" model, the "seesaw" is broken, but there is no extension of the analogy. In the "brake and accelerator" model, this is like driving a car with a foot on the brakes and accelerator at the same time. This helps to explain the situation much more fully, as you will see.

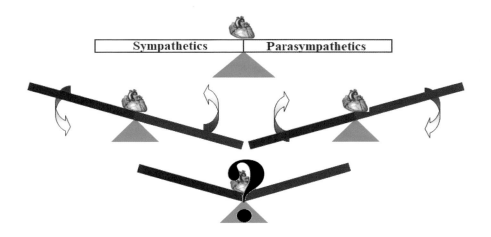

## Introduction

A failure of the proper interaction between P&S leads to disorder and possibly disease. To extend the analogy, if you do not take your foot off the brakes and hit the accelerator, you still go, but you must use much more gas (again, read that as "adrenaline") and you must over-rev your engine (read that as "overstimulate the Sympathetics") to go anywhere. This places more wear on the engine (the heart, kidneys, and body) and on the brakes (the Parasympathetics). The problem is, in the human, once the "brakes" (the Parasympathetics) wear out, they cannot be replaced. Eventually you will roll down a hill and "crash." This could lead to an acute vascular event in older patients (the heart attack or stroke) or severe fatigue, light-headedness, pain, and headache in younger patients.

In clinical terms at this point, your Parasympathetics are not strong enough to prevent a sympathetically mediated Ventricular tachyrhythm from becoming fibrillation, which may lead to a heart attack. Therefore, therapy is based on "getting your foot off the brakes" (reducing Parasympathetic activity) to minimize wear on the "brakes" and the "engine." This may include anticholinergic therapy, also known as very low-dose antidepressant therapy; on the order of $1/10^{th}$ the traditional dose of antidepressants.

Therapy may also target the Sympathetics as secondary in order to minimize cardiovascular stress as the two autonomic branches are normalizing. This secondary, Sympathetic therapy may be needed to protect the systems during the healing process. Think of it this way. Remember the P&S nervous systems are independent systems. Therefore, if the Sympathetics are in the "habit" of over-revving the engine, this may continue for a while, even though you are removing your foot from the brakes. This will cause the car to speed up even more at first (read that HR or BP to go even higher). This is the result of the "bad habit" (Dysautonomia) of compensating for your foot being on the brakes. Until the Sympathetics are habituated to "less brakes," therapy will be needed to prevent further harm.

"Over-revving your engine" which is exaggerating, or overstimulating, your stress responses (Sympathetic responses), explains the symptoms of Anxiety. In Anxiety, due to Parasympathetic Excess, small worries are amplified into large worries, which may become mentally crippling. If pain is involved, small touches become very painful responses. Instead of the Parasympathetics decreasing, they increase (Parasympathetic Excess or PE), forcing the Sympathetics to increase that much further to generate the same response (see Figure 1). This is the "amplification" process. Similarly in pain syndromes, normal stimuli (light touch and tickle) are amplified into pain responses, and significant pain response may become physically crippling. This helps to explain diffuse pain syndromes such as fibromyalgia and difficult-to-manage pain syndromes such as Chronic Regional Pain Syndrome. Again, assuming no end organ effects, relieving the PE alone will eventually relieve the Sympathetic Excess (SE), which eventually relieves the symptoms.

To further extend the car analogy, as you are driving along, and everything is calm, what is your first reaction to a sudden, unexpected, event? . . . You hit the brakes. This is a protective response. Hitting the "brakes" or "riding the brakes" explains the symptoms of addiction. Again, your body is very similar. The "brakes" (the Parasympathetics) are the protective mechanism. In addition, the "brakes" cause the patient to seek their "comfort zone" (safety), whether it be drugs, alcohol, sex, food, or whatever is their compulsion. The Parasympathetics are strongly associated with the "Pleasure Centers" or "Comfort  Centers" of the brain stem. Once addicted, the Parasympathetics tend to remain excessive. If the PE is not relieved during rehabilitation, then the risk of relapse

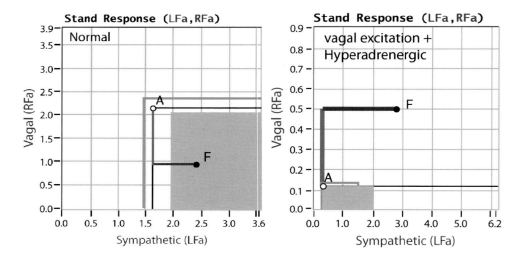

**Figure 1**: The normal response (left graph), as exemplified in the P&S response to standing (F) from sitting (A), is the Parasympathetics (the blue line) decreasing first, followed by the Sympathetics (the red line) increasing. Removing the foot from the brakes, then accelerating, minimizes the amount of acceleration required and potentiates the effects of acceleration. The abnormal situation of "riding the brakes" (right graph), is the Parasympathetics (the blue line) increasing forcing the Sympathetics (the red line) to increase further, thereby "over-revving" the engine. Therapy should target removing the patient's foot from the brakes (Parasympathetics). This typically, organically, reduces the amount of acceleration (Sympathetics), assuming no end-organ effects.

remains high due to the excessive (Parasympathetic) drive in the patient to remain in their "comfort zone" stimulating their "pleasure centers."

"Riding the brakes" helps to explain other common symptoms. One is "brain fog" and cognitive and memory difficulties: PE acts to limit the output of the heart under stress. This results in poor brain profusion, which results in reduced brain activity, similar to that associated with depression. Another common symptom is fatigue. Often, patients describe their fatigue as if they were "running a marathon while sitting still." Again, PE will cause this by causing normal responses to little, normal stresses to be amplified into excessive responses. A minor activity becomes a major undertaking, increasing cardiac function, metabolism, and energy expenditure while doing little if anything.

A third common symptom is sleep difficulty. If you take more than twenty minutes to fall asleep, or wake more than twice a night (even to go to the bathroom), then your sleep difficulty may be caused by PE. Consider what happens when a patient faints. Besides gravity working, once flat on the ground, the heart and head are at the same level. The brain is receiving all the blood it wants; it's happy, but the patient is not. Similarly, after being upright all day (sitting or standing), as soon as the patient lies down to go to sleep, their brain (which has been partially asleep all day) now has all the blood it wants; it wants to play, the patient wants to sleep. The patient typically lies there processing their day, reviewing lists of things to do, and planning for the morrow. The patient may also rise frequently during the night (more than twice) even to go to the bathroom, because the brain is active (the brain makes you feel like you have to go to the bathroom, but really it just wants to go for a ride, so you may sit there and nothing happens). Restoring proper brain profusion (blood flow to the brain) will "wake up" the brain, process the day, and then, with the normal brain changes with evening, the brain will be ready for sleep at the same time as the patient.

In general, PE is associated with the following (in no order of importance or frequency): difficult-to-control BP, blood glucose, weight, or hormone level, difficult-to-describe pain syndromes (including CRPS), difficult-to-manage weight loss, unexplained arrhythmia (palpitations) or seizure, and symptoms of depression or anxiety, fatigue, exercise intolerance, sex dysfunction, sleep or GI disturbance, light-headedness, cognitive dysfunction or "brain fog," or frequent headache or migraine.

P&S monitoring provides more information. It is a simple, noninvasive, quick, inexpensive study that may easily be performed in the clinic in about fifteen minutes. It is the only noninvasive technology that quantifies Parasympathetic activity, independent of, and simultaneously with, Sympathetic activity. All other noninvasive autonomic technologies force assumption and approximation to theorize P&S activity. P&S monitoring technology was developed in animal models through the 1980s with chemical, electrical, and mechanical blockade studies [31–34]. By the early 1990s, P&S monitoring was verified and validated in humans. Both the animal and early human studies were performed at MIT and Harvard Medical School. The majority of the human studies were performed at beta-sites throughout the United States, including Harvard, Cleveland Clinic, the University of Pennsylvania, Stanford University, and fourteen others. P&S monitoring was USFDA cleared in 1995, and US Medicare accepted in 1997. It continues to be patented and well published in numerous journals of many clinical disciplines.

The P&S nervous systems are the brain-heart, or more generally,

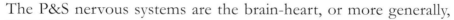

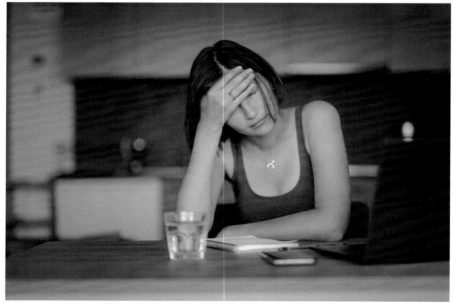

the mind-body connection. P&S monitoring is more information about the physiologic condition of the individual patient. It also has ramifications regarding the mental health of the individual as well as provides data regarding brain perfusion and sleep function. Typically, if a patient is monitored early, the P&S information is earlier than other physiologic measures. Remember, the P&S nervous system controls the organs, and its purpose is to maintain normal organ function even when it, itself, is abnormal. Ultimately, Dysautonomia (abnormal P&S function) will be translated to the organ system or systems. As an aside, this is why there is usually an onset latency to post-trauma syndromes, for example, or autonomic dysfunction in pre-diabetes or even metabolic syndrome, long before diabetes is diagnosed. Also, given that the P&S nervous systems are the repositories of the individual patient's health history, including the memory for the immune system (which is why vaccines are helpful), we may state that P&S monitoring documents the patient's individual and specific "physiologic fingerprint."

P&S monitoring provides more information to healthcare providers throughout the fields of healthcare and beyond, including chronic care, critical care, mental health, assisted living (including nursing homes), and wellness programs. The more information helps providers to reduce morbidity and mortality risk and reduce medication load, and therefore reduce hospitalization and re-hospitalization, all the while improving patient outcomes and reducing costs.

P&S monitoring independently and simultaneously quantifies both autonomic systems. As published in a recent, leading cardiology journal, all other noninvasive, autonomic, single beat-to-beat cardiac measures are not sufficient to characterize P&S activity [35]. P&S monitoring is the most useful [2]. With P&S monitoring, it is not necessary to default to invasive neural testing to get more precise quantitative data in more benign autonomic dysfunction situations, especially if it is not a life-threatening condition. All other noninvasive autonomic measures are based on only the one beat-to-beat measure of the heart and therefore are only a measure of total autonomic function. The other autonomic measures are, therefore, ambiguous and force assumption and approximation to theorize P&S activity.

P&S monitoring provides more information for chronic care medicine, which typically is the majority of national healthcare costs. P&S guided therapy often relieves multiple symptoms at the same time, rather than only treating the individual symptoms in isolation. Furthermore, if there are no end-organ deficits, P&S-guided therapy is often not lifelong. In these cases, it is possible to "retrain" the P&S systems (like breaking a bad habit and establishing and stabilizing a good habit). Once stabilized, the P&S systems may carry forward on their own without the help of therapy until some other clinical event occurs. To this end, if a condition is detected early enough, before symptoms, P&S therapy is preventative and short-term (nine to eighteen months).

Ultimately, chronic disease, like Anxiety, accelerates the onset of autonomic dysfunction including cardiovascular autonomic neuropathy (CAN, defined as very low, resting Parasympathetic activity and is late-, to end-stage autonomic dysfunction). In summary, P&S guided therapy reduces morbidity and mortality risks, reduces medication load, improves patient outcomes, and reduces costs.

To test the P&S nervous systems, a multiphased test is necessary, primarily due to the fact that the P&S systems are dynamic systems. Most medical tests are not dynamic, patients are at rest (sitting or supine) when tested. The P&S nervous systems are never resting. Even when you are asleep the nervous system is active, arguably more active than when you are awake. Therefore, typically, patients are tested, diagnosed, and treated to normalize their resting state. Unfortunately, most Dysautonomias are not demonstrated while at rest. Therefore, a dynamic test must be administered. Another need for a dynamic P&S test is that a patient is seen only periodically by a physician. Information representing the patient's responses when not in the physician's office helps to better manage the patient. However, it is also helpful to be able to diagnose and initiate therapy on the first test.

The resulting test is a fifteen minute, thirty-five second test:

A. The first five minutes is a resting baseline that enables the patient to become their own control, enabling same-day diagnosis and therapy.

B. Deep or Paced Breathing at six breaths per minute for a minute. Six breaths per minute is the average optimal stimulus for the human Parasympathetic nervous system. Deep Breathing simulates patient responses to disease and therapy after large meals, before bedtime, and other Parasympathetic-dominant situations.

C. The patient is then returned to baseline and normal breathing for a minute.

D. The Valsalva challenge is five short Valsalva maneuvers, with intervening rest periods over a minute and thirty-five seconds. Valsalva maneuvers simulate patient responses to disease and therapy during stress, exercise, and other Sympathetic dominant situations. This includes the standard fifteen-second Valsalva and helps to document baroreceptor reflex function.

E. The patient is then returned to baseline and normal breathing for two minutes.

F. The last five minutes include a quick change from sitting to standing or tilt. Either way, it is a head-up postural change challenge. In fact, this portion of the test largely replaces a tilt test [36]. The stand challenge is important for documenting the causes of light-headedness. It is also important for documenting the coordination between the P&S nervous systems. If they do not coordinate properly (as in the "brake and accelerator" analogy) for something as common as standing, they may not be coordinating the organs properly. Which organ is significantly affected is determined based on symptoms or further testing as needed, given the patient's medical history.

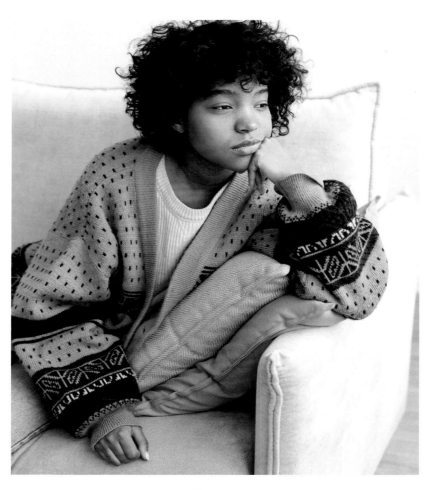

## TESTING PROCEDURE

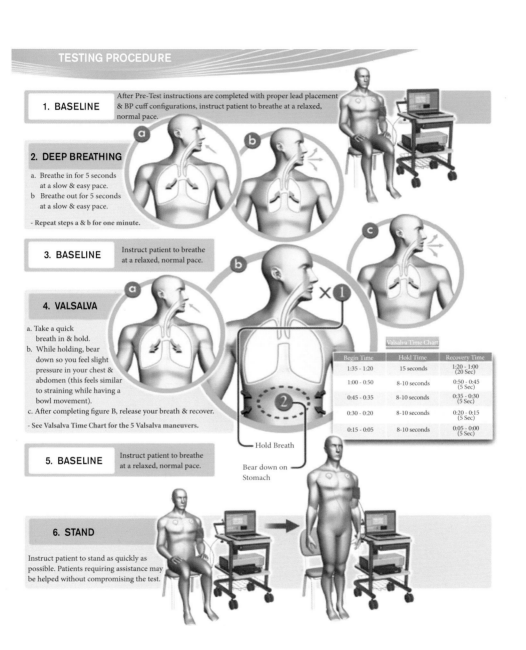

**1. BASELINE** — After Pre-Test instructions are completed with proper lead placement & BP cuff configurations, instruct patient to breathe at a relaxed, normal pace.

**2. DEEP BREATHING**

a. Breathe in for 5 seconds at a slow & easy pace.
b. Breathe out for 5 seconds at a slow & easy pace.

- Repeat steps a & b for one minute.

**3. BASELINE** — Instruct patient to breathe at a relaxed, normal pace.

**4. VALSALVA**

a. Take a quick breath in & hold.
b. While holding, bear down so you feel slight pressure in your chest & abdomen (this feels similar to straining while having a bowl movement).
c. After completing figure B, release your breath & recover.

- See Valsalva Time Chart for the 5 Valsalva maneuvers.

Valsalva Time Chart

| Begin Time | Hold Time | Recovery Time |
|---|---|---|
| 1:35 - 1:20 | 15 seconds | 1:20 - 1:00 (20 Sec) |
| 1:00 - 0:50 | 8-10 seconds | 0:50 - 0:45 (5 Sec) |
| 0:45 - 0:35 | 8-10 seconds | 0:35 - 0:30 (5 Sec) |
| 0:30 - 0:20 | 8-10 seconds | 0:20 - 0:15 (5 Sec) |
| 0:15 - 0:05 | 8-10 seconds | 0:05 - 0:00 (5 Sec) |

Hold Breath

Bear down on Stomach

**5. BASELINE** — Instruct patient to breathe at a relaxed, normal pace.

**6. STAND**

Instruct patient to stand as quickly as possible. Patients requiring assistance may be helped without compromising the test.

If the patient is a wheelchair user, and cannot stand for even a couple of minutes, then the entire test may be performed supine and the patient either quickly tilted (if a tilt table) and remain tilted for the five minutes, or requested to quickly sit up and remain with proper seated posture for the five minutes.

None of these challenges should cause symptoms. While the patient should not talk during the test, if there are symptoms, even if they are mild, the patient should let the technician know immediately. The reason is that symptoms may be more revealing than borderline results. To this end, the test is still valid even if the patient cannot complete some of the challenges. If symptoms are significant, then abort the challenge and, if need be, reseat the patient and finish the challenge, then continue the rest of the test. To minimize artifact, there should also be no moving during the test, unless otherwise directed.

Unless directed by your physician, do not change or alter your therapy protocol or your typical lifestyle. It takes the nervous system up to three months to fully adapt to a change in therapy or lifestyle. Therefore, a short-term (one- or two-day) change will not have a significant effect.

Please avoid a significant meal within half an hour of testing or a significant exercise period within an hour of testing. In this case, significant exercise may include climbing a flight of stairs if the patient has heart failure, for example.

The test will require you to have three EKG electrodes placed on your chest and a blood pressure cuff placed on your arm. For comfort and convenience, wear a two-piece outfit, with no body lotions, oils, or sprays.

# Disclaimers

Drs. DePace and Colombo are the authors of the book upon which this is based:

DePace NL, Colombo J. *Autonomic and Mitochondrial Dysfunction in Clinical Diseases: Diagnostic, Prevention, and Therapy.*
Springer Science + Business Media, New York, NY, 2019.

While we have developed the supplement package described as part of the Mind-Body Wellness Program, all of these supplements are readily available through common commercial means (i.e., your neighborhood pharmacy).

Drs. DePace and Colombo are some of the authors of the book upon which the implementation and application of P&S monitoring is based:

Colombo J, Arora RR, DePace NL, Vinik AI.
*Clinical Autonomic Dysfunction: Measurement, Indications, Therapies, and Outcomes.*
Springer Science + Business Media, New York, NY, 2014.

Drs. DePace and Colombo are co-owners of the research organization from which some of the data included herein was collected and analyzed: NeuroCardiology Research Corporation.

Dr. Colombo is a co-owner, Chief Technology Officer, and Senior Medical Director of Physio PS, Inc., the producer and provider of P&S monitoring technologies.

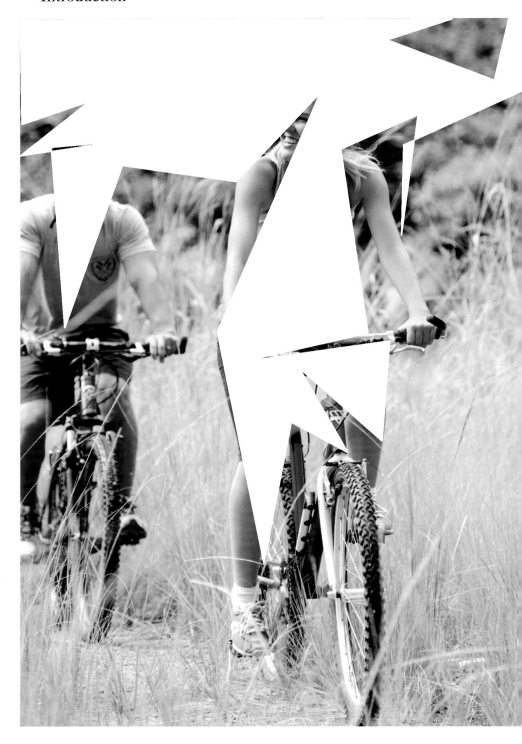

The information and contents, including medical information, in this book are solely and strictly offered as an educational and informational resource. The use of this book shall be expressly limited as an informational tool to help improve awareness and understanding of Dysautonomia in fatigue syndromes for both patients and physicians. This book is not intended to, and does not claim to, provide any medical or professional advice or diagnosis, or medical or professional opinion, or medical or professional treatment services of any kind, whether pharmaceutical, supplemental, nutraceutical, or lifestyle, to any individual. This book shall in no way substitute or replace the patient-physicial relationship or be used as a substitute for medical or professional diagnosis and treatment. Please consult a board-certified physician for medical advice or treatment and before making any decisions or changes in your healthcare treatment plan(s).

*We wish all a lifetime of happiness and wellness. Enjoy!*

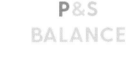

# CHRONIC FATIGUE SYNDROME

## Diagnosis

ME/CFS is a clinical diagnosis that can be made only when other etiologies of fatigue have been excluded. Specific diagnostic criteria for CFS were developed by the Centers for Disease Control and Prevention (CDC) in 1988. During this time, it was theorized that viral illness was the primary etiology of CFS; therefore, the criteria focused on physical symptoms. To parallel the World Health Organization categorization of CFS as a neurologic disorder, the Oxford criteria were developed in 1991 (Table 1). These criteria emphasize mental fatigue over physical symptoms [37]. Table 2 lists the possible symptoms of CFS and the P or S branch of the nervous system that is associated with that symptom. The CDC's

**Table 1:** Oxford Criteria for Chronic Fatigue Syndrome [37].
*All criteria must be met to make the diagnosis.*

- Primary symptom is fatigue.
- Definite onset of symptoms.
- Fatigue is severe, disabling, and affects physical and mental functioning.
- Symptoms for at least six months and present more than 50 percent of the time.
- Other symptoms must be present, particularly myalgia and mood and sleep disturbances.
- Certain patients should be excluded:
  - Those with an established medical condition known to produce chronic fatigue;
  - Those with a current diagnosis of schizophrenia, manic-depressive illness, substance abuse, eating disorder, or proven organic brain disease.

# DEAR PATIENT
# OR
# THE LOVED ONE OF A PATIENT

# CHRONIC FATIGUE SYNDROME

## Diagnosis

You must know that there is no diagnostic test that is accurate enough to prove that a person has CFS. It is extremely import- ant to avoid the controversy of whether this is psychogenic or an organic symptom or whether it is caused by infection. For in fact, in any one individual's case, it may be due to all or some or only one of these. That is why, if you read what we say to the physi- cian, you see that many tests are needed to rule out ME/CFS. That is not to say that you do not have fatigue. Indeed, you may have fatigue. It may be what we call "persistent fatigue" as it is associ- ated with many other diseases. Understanding the difference and perhaps helping your physician to understand the difference will help lead to the proper therapy for you. More information is good in this case, but it has to be the correct information and interpreted properly. To help with gathering more information, we will also introduce P&S monitoring as an added test to help gather more information and to track the progression of your specific disorder and your responses to treatment(s).

**Table 2**: ME/CFS Symptoms and branch of the Autonomic Nervous System (P or S) that may affect the symptom. [Adapted from 38]

| FREQUENT SYMPTOMS | P or S |
|---|---|
| Debilitating fatigue greater than 6 months | P |
| Sore throat | P,S |
| Swollen glands and tender Lymph nodes | P,S |
| Diarrhea | P |

**Table 3:** Centers for Disease Control and Prevention Diagnostic Criteria for Chronic Fatigue Syndrome [38].

---

Severe fatigue for longer than six (6) months, and at least four (4) of the following symptoms:

- Headache of new type, pattern, or severity;
- Multi-joint pain without swelling or erythema;
- Muscle pain;
- Post-exertional malaise for longer than twenty-four hours;
- Significant impairment in short-term memory or concentration;
- Sore throat;
- Tender lymph nodes; or
- Unrefreshing sleep.

---

criteria were revised in 1994 to broaden the definition, and at this time, are the most widely accepted diagnostic criteria for CFS (Table 3).

The general approach to a patient with CFS should start with a history and physical examination, focusing on identifying the most bothersome symptoms and red flag symptoms (Table 4) that may indicate a more serious underlying illness based on the National Institute for Health and Clinical Excellence (NICE) guidelines. Patients should have a mental status examination, including evaluation for depression, which is present in 39 percent to 47 percent of patients with CFS.* Although the differential diagnosis for patients presenting with CFS is broad (Table 5), approximately one-third meet the

---

\* Although Depression may not only be a psychiatric issue, many with depression also have a P or S dysfunction that causes poor brain perfusion which often leads to depression and fatigue.

**Table 2**: (continued)

| | |
|---|---|
| Fatigue after exertion | P |
| Muscle aches and pains | S |
| Joint pain | S |
| Fever | P,S |
| Chills | P |
| Unrefreshing sleep | P |
| Sleep difficulties | P |
| Headaches | P,S |
| Memory or Cognitive Difficulties | P |
| "Brain Fog" (lack of concentration) | P |
| Nausea | P |
| Stomach or Abdominal pain | P |
| Sinus or Nasal problems | P,S |
| Shortness of breath | P,S |
| Sensitivity to light | P,S |
| Depression | P |

**Table 4**: Red Flag Symptoms in Persons with Suspected Chronic Fatigue Syndrome [39].

| RED FLAGS | DISEASE PROCESS INDICATED |
|---|---|
| Chest pain | Cardiac disease |
| Focal neurologic deficits | Central nervous system malignancy or abscess, multiple sclerosis |
| Inflammatory signs or joint pain | Autoimmune disease (e.g., rheumatoid arthritis, systemic lupus erythematosus) |
| Lymphadenopathy or weight loss | Malignancy |
| Shortness of breath | Pulmonary disease |

criteria for CFS. No laboratory tests can be used to diagnose CFS; instead, they are used to rule out other causes of fatigue[†] that would preclude the diagnosis of CFS. The CDC and NICE recommend a minimal set of tests for patients presenting with CFS.

The CDC recommends initial evaluation with urinalysis; complete blood count; comprehensive metabolic panel; and measurements of phosphorus, thyroid-stimulating hormone, and C-reactive protein. NICE also recommends using ten months of immunoglobulin A endomysial antibodies to screen for celiac disease, and, if indicated by the history or physical examination, urine drug screening, rheumatoid factor testing, and antinuclear antibody testing. Viral titers are not recommended unless the patient's history is suggestive of an infectious process, because they do not confirm or eliminate the diagnosis of CFS.

---

† These may include Lyme disease, fibromyalgia, and Autoimmune Disorders, however, we believe that these are actually disorders of the P&S nervous systems. Lyme disease is killed by the antibiotic prescribed, however, the lingering symptoms that escalate are due to prolonged oxidative stress that continues to damage cells and ultimately leads to systemic disorders. Fibromyalgia (and some other myalgias) are generalized pain syndromes that are due to a hidden Parasympathetic Excess (PE see below) that amplifies Sympathetic responses to touch, causing them to be pain responses. This PE may also include Small Fiber Disease which is characterized by inflammation of the pain and autonomic nerve fibers. Autoimmune Disorders are also likely to be due to PE that causes the immune system to be overactive and over-activated and as a result turning on the healthy tissue of the body that resembles whatever foreign entity it that portion of the immune system was designed to attack. A reason why many autoimmune disorders are neurological is because the myelin sheathing of nerves often resembles the protein coats of viruses.

All of the symptoms in Table 3 must be experienced frequently for six (6) months or more for ME/CFS to be diagnosed. Anything short of this we would classify as persistent fatigue. From P&S monitoring, most of the symptoms listed in Table 2 are known to be associated with Parasympathetic Excess that occurs during a Sympathetic or Stress challenge (PE) [23]. Those that are not known to be associated with PE (i.e., the symptoms marked with "P,S") may be explained by PE.

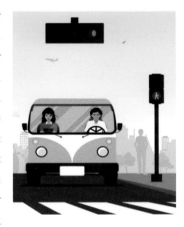

PE may be understood if you consider the P&S nervous systems like the brakes and accelerator, respectively, on a car (with an automatic transmission). When stopped at a red light with your foot on the brakes, what is the first thing you do when the light turns green? . . . You take your foot off the brakes. Even before you touch the accelerator, the car begins to roll. You are already accelerating. By taking your foot off the brakes, you minimize the amount of gas you need to begin to move, and you minimize wear on the engine needed to accelerate. This keeps the engine's revolutions per minute (RPMs) low. To facilitate this, your brakes also work faster than your accelerator. This is important, because if it were the other way, you may never stop if the brakes could not catch up to the accelerator. By the way, this is essentially how a heart attack happens.

Your body is very similar. Normally, when you are ready to move (including sitting or standing up) or react to something (physically, mentally, or emotionally), the Parasympathetics (your "brakes") first decrease, then the Sympathetics (your "accelerator") increase. This minimizes the amount of adrenaline (the "gas" in the autonomic

**Table 5**: Differential Diagnosis of Chronic Fatigue, given below as nine (9) separate lists.

| ENDOCRINE | HEMATOLOGIC/ ONCOLOGIC |
|---|---|
| Addison disease | Anemia |
| Adrenal insufficiency | Malignancy |
| Cushing disease | **INFECTIOUS** |
| Diabetes mellitus | Chronic hepatitis |
| Hyperthyroidism | Human immunodeficiency virus |
| Hypothyroidism | Lyme disease |
| **NEUROLOGIC** | Tuberculosis |
| Dementia | **PSYCHIATRIC** |
| Multiple Sclerosis | Depression and Anxiety |
| Narcolepsy | Depression–Anxiety Syndromes |
| Insomnia | Eating Disorders |
| Parkinson's Disease | Major Depressive Disorder |
| **CARDIOLOGY** | Schizophrenia |
| Poor oxygenation of red blood cells | Somatoform Disorders |
| Poor circulation | Substance Abuse |
| Arrhythmias | **PULMONOLOGY** |
| Blocked arteries | Shortness of breath |
| Heart Failure | Poor oxygen exchange in the lungs |
| Defective heart valves | **OTHERS** |
| **RHEUMATOLOGIC** | Obesity |
| Dermatomyositis | Malnutrition |
| Fibromyalgia | Psychosocial Stress |
| Hypermobility (EDS) | Allergies |
| Collagen Vascular Disease | Chronic Pain |
|  | Orthostatic Dysfunction |
|  | Syncope |

EDS: Ehlers-Danlos Syndrome, the genetic form of hypermobility.

system) you need to begin to move, and you minimize your stress reaction (wear on the engine as measured by RPMs) you need to accelerate.

If, however, you do not remove your foot from the brakes before stepping on the accelerator, you still go, but it requires you to over-rev your engine (it requires many more RPMs to move). In your body, it requires much more energy to act or react to the same stimuli. This is the beginning of fatigue. Keeping your foot on the brakes is called "riding the brakes." This is like PE. PE forces the Sympathetics to overreact, causing Sympathetic Excess (SE). PE causes small stimuli to be overamplified: little touches become painful, little concerns become anxiety, what should be little energy expenditures become excessive and fatiguing. Pain and anxiety, in general excess energy expenditures, are associated with SE.

The problem with PE is twofold. First, few doctors know that the Parasympathetics may be measured, therefore, they do not know that PE is possible. Second, the SE (caused by PE) is the only thing a that doctor may see (remember, they do not know that the Parasympathetics can be measured). SE causes high heart rate and high blood pressure and is associated with shortness of breath and pain, as well as inflammation and oxidative stress (like in sore throats and swollen glands). As a result, your doctors feel justified in treating the SE as the primary disorder. However, this usually makes the PE worse and, therefore, makes the SE worse because the body has more ways to increase Sympathetic activity than medicine has ways to block these increases. Since you do not respond as expected, your doctors begin to question whether you are complying with the therapy plan, and eventually, they question whether

There has been some literature that suggests that controlling P&S symptoms can improve function in CFS and effective trials of medications to treat P&S symptoms should be pursued. Studies have shown that functional ability or disability in CFS has been better predicted by P&S dysfunction [40,41]. Orthostatic hypotension is a common P&S symptom and, as a result, a common feature of many chronic diseases, including CFS [42]. As mentioned above, POTS is another orthostatic dysfunction. POTS is a disorder of orthostatic intolerance involving an increase in HR of greater than 30 bpm above the baseline without a drop in BP (without orthostatic hypotension).

In POTS, growing evidence suggests an association with CFS. In one small study, nearly one-third of the participants with CFS presented with a diagnosis of POTS based on hemodynamic testing [43]. Another small study found that 93 percent of the group had symptoms of severe fatigue and fulfilled criteria for CFS when assessing patients with POTS [44].

# PERSISTENT FATIGUE

Chronic Fatigue Syndrome (CFS) addressed in the previous section is a specific diagnosis for which the majority of fatigue patients do not qualify. "Persistent" fatigue (as it is defined in this book) is differentiated from CFS [45] to be able to better address the symptoms of fatigue. Mitochondrial dysfunction and P&S dysfunction are considered to be biological mechanisms of fatigue. An autoimmune basis is still being investigated. Fatigue is described as a lack of energy and mental or physical tiredness, diminished endurance, and prolonged recovery after physical activity, but it has to be persistent and continuous for at least six months: therefore "chronic fatigue." What do patients do in the meantime?

you are truly experiencing these symptoms or if they are only in your head. You know that they are not in your head. This is when the relationship breaks down and you are left to suffer.

P&S monitoring documents that PE is real, how it is expressed in you, personally, and thereby how to best treat it. By relieving PE, SE will eventually be relieved, which will then eventually relieve high heart rates and blood pressures and excessive pain responses and inflammation. Given the title of this book, relieving the Dysautonomia and PE, and establishing P&S balance relieves the associated fatigue (whether chronic or persistent) and eventually the associated symptoms. Once P&S balance is established, any remaining symptoms (including fatigue) may be due to organ damage within the body. This organ damage may require continued therapy. Either way, maintaining P&S balance helps to establish and maintain wellness.

Table 5 includes a list of diagnoses that may include fatigue, but preclude CFS. Typically treating these diseases or disorders also helps to relieve the fatigue. However, overtreating them may also cause fatigue, so you need to be careful and work with your physician to avoid fatigue.

# PERSISTENT FATIGUE

Most people do not fit the diagnosis of Chronic Fatigue Syndrome, yet they have significant or even debilitating fatigue. To help you to receive support and healthcare attention, we are classifying these people as suffering persistent fatigue. Included in the persistent fatigue classification are all of the people who to do qualify as CFS due to another disease or disorder, including, but not limited to: depression, Lyme's disease, fibromyalgia, chronic pain, heart disease, arrhythmia, chronic kidney disease, pulmonary disorders

As physicians, do we simply let them suffer until the criteria are met? What if not all criteria are met? What do we do then? We are trained to reduce suffering. This process does not achieve that goal, especially when there are things that may be implemented to help immediately.

Mitochondrial dysfunction, including deficits in mitochondrial enzymes and excesses in oxidative or nitrosative stresses, have been implicated as causes of deficits in mitochondrial energy metabolism and Adenosine Tri-Phosphate (ATP, the "energy molecule") production from fatty acid metabolism. Mitochondria have an essential role in energy production from oxidative phosphorylation of electrons into ATP, which powers the activities of most cells.

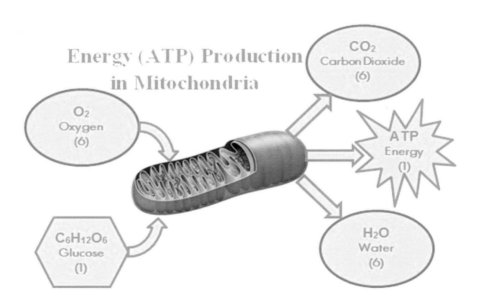

(including COPD, cystic fibrosis, and emphysema), advanced diabetes, advanced Parkinson's, dementia, anorexia-bulimia, anxiety, GI disorders that cause malnutrition, mitochondrial disorder, chronic mast cell disorder, sleep disorders (both too little sleep and too much sleep), chronic immune disorders, some hormonal disorders, syncope, orthostatic dysfunction (including orthostatic hypotension and postural orthostatic tachycardia syndrome), collagen vascular diseases (EDS and the hypermobility spectrum diseases), and more. Some of these are recognized as being associated with fatigue, but many are not or are not well understood. Unfortunately, many fatigue patients must inform their healthcare providers, rather than the other way around.

At the root of many of these disorders is either or both mitochondrial disorder or autonomic (P&S) disorder. We know that mitochondrial disorder may lead to P&S disorder. We suspect that

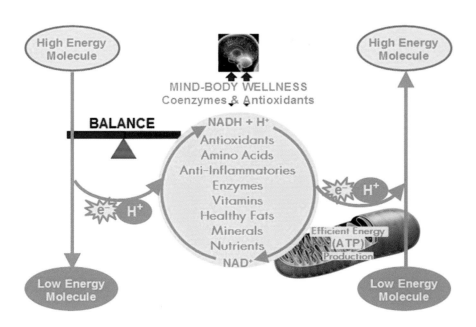

The antioxidant coenzyme Q10 is the most commonly investigated mitochondrial enzyme. Low levels of CoQ10 were consistently associated with fatigue [46]. However, like most things in life, there needs to be a proper balance. In the healthy state, mitochondria are the largest producers of oxidants in the human body, specifically the oxidants known as reactive oxygen species (ROS[‡]). Low, or physiological, levels of ROS are signaling molecules within the mitochondria to modulate mitochondrial function and coordinate mitochondrial function with the functions of the cells they are in, in a beneficial way [47]; and they are in most cells of the body.[§]

Being the largest producer of oxidants in the body sounds counter-intuitive; however, low levels of oxidants are need for healthy function. In addition to the signaling process mentioned above, oxidants are especially important for the immune system. Oxidation of detritus and invading or foreign species (e.g., bacteria, viruses, and molds) is a first line of defense within the body.

So a proper antioxidant-oxidant balance is necessary for health and wellness [48]. CoQ10 is arguably one of the two most powerful antioxidants naturally made by your body. The other is alpha-lipoic acid. These two are not only the strongest, in and of themselves, but they are made stronger still because they recycle other antioxidants within the body, like vitamins A, C, and E. For example, vitamin C, on the one hand is said to be harmful because it may

---

‡  In small amounts, these ROS are beneficial in "burning the trash" (waste products and worn membranes) and helping the immune systems to "burn-out" invaders attempting to make one sick.

§  Neurons (including brain cells) and cardiomyocytes (heart cells) both of which effect the entire body, have the highest concentrations of mitochondria due to their high energy needs.

P&S disorder may lead to mitochondrial disorder. The reason why we know that mitochondrial disorder may lead to P&S is because the nerves (along with the heart) are the largest consumers of energy in the body and, to that end, have the largest number of mitochondria per cell in the body. We suspect that P&S disorder may lead to mitochondrial disorder because the P&S nervous systems control or coordinate every cell in the body and to do so may modulate mitochondrial activity.

In addition to generating the energy molecule of the body (ATP), mitochondria also generate oxidants. This sounds counterproductive, since most know that oxidants cause illness and stress and can lead to fatigue; but it is not. In fact, like most things in life, a proper balance is healthy, including for antioxidants and oxidants.

All things are used for good (little goes to waste) in the body, including "bad" things. Oxidation is a form of burning. Oxidants are used in the body for many different functions. For example, oxidation of carbon (as in wood or paper) is what is commonly known as fire. In this way, oxidants are used to "burn" as in a fire, to help generate heat. Oxidants are used to burn "trash," as in cells that have worn out and have been replaced. Another important use of oxidants is by the immune system, where immune cells collect oxidants as "burning coals" and use them to "torch" invading bacteria, viruses, molds, mildews, debris and other unwanted things. Every time we breathe in, swallow, or absorb something through the skin (let alone break the skin), we take in a myriad of unwanted and harmful things and the immune system uses oxidants, among other things, together with the micro-organisms that symbiotically live within us, to eliminate invaders before they can make us sick.

burn in the urine (and possibly damage the glomeruli in the kidneys), and on the other hand it is nearly considered a panacea. The reason for this is that the studies that are used to support these claims do not control for these most powerful antioxidants: alpha-lipoic acid (ALA) and coenzyme Q10 (CoQ10). These most powerful antioxidants recycle the other antioxidants and make them more powerful as well, thereby making themselves more powerful in the process. Without healthy levels of ALA or CoQ10, then the other antioxidants are not recycled and are not very helpful. In the vitamin C example, with low levels of ALA and CoQ10, vitamin C gets only one pass through the body (the bloodstream). In this case, since vitamin C gets only one pass through the body and is immediately filtered out of the blood by the kidneys, the resulting concentration in the kidneys and then the urine is high, and vitamin C may burn if taken in high doses. With healthy levels of ALA or CoQ10, vitamin C is recycled, has more opportunities to be effective as an antioxidant, and, in the process, is diluted in the kidneys and does not burn. This is an example of the reason why published opinions on these vitamins and other antioxidants range from harmful to most helpful.

All in all, a proper antioxidant-oxidant balance is required to restore and maintain health and wellness. In effect, this has been proven in the negative [49]. With mitochondria dysfunction, not only is ATP production low, but oxidant production is low. Then, not only are there not enough energy molecules (ATP) available to overcome fatigue and "brain fog" and the like, but the immune system is less effective and people tend to be sicker, including with sore throats and swollen lymph glands. Conditions such as hypermobility and Ehlers-Danlos Syndrome (EDS) cause the body's connective tissue to be loose and "leaky," and the oxidant levels must be much higher.

If the mitochondria are "sick" and antioxidant production is low, then not only are there not enough energy molecules (ATP) available to overcome fatigue and "brain fog" and the like, but our immune system is less effective and we tend to be sicker, including with sore throats and swollen lymph glands. Conditions such as hypermobility and Ehlers-Danlos Syndrome (EDS), cause the body's connective tissue to be loose and "leaky," and the oxidant levels must be much higher. The connective tissue forms a barrier to prevent things from "leaking in" as well. Without this barrier, the immune system is even more active than usual 24/7, contributing to fatigue. In cancer therapy, specifically chemotherapy, oxidants are purposely introduced into the body to help destroy the cancer. This is why chemo patients may not be permitted to take antioxidants. You should consult your physician.

Just like most other things, too much of a good thing is still not good. Too many oxidants will destroy mitochondria, as well as other important tissues. So a proper antioxidant-oxidant balance is important. The production of oxidants by the mitochondria is

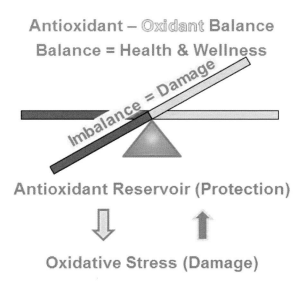

The connective tissue forms a barrier to prevent things from "leaking in" as well as "leaking out." As a result, the immune system is overactive trying to prevent illness, and in the process, needs many more oxidants to burn out things that should not be in the body. This begins the process of fatigue in cases of hypermobility and EDS.

Fatigue is the hallmark of mitochondrial dysfunction. Alterations in energy and metabolism may contribute to fatigue. Many of these studies were cross-sectional and only studied patients with CFS, and the findings were inconsistent between mitochondrial biomarkers and fatigue, suggesting that it may not have all been chronic fatigue. Antioxidants were not always controlled. Reduced levels of CoQ10, known to increase ROS levels, have been found in some studies. Increased levels of ROS with decreased levels of antioxidants have been found in other studies. [1]

Mitochondrial dysfunction may be a differentiating marker between CFS and fibromyalgia [50], another disorder known to include persistent fatigue more than CFS, specifically. Mitochondrial dysfunction is significantly lower in fibromyalgia patients but not in CFS patients. Also, mitochondrial DNA content was normal with CFS patients and reduced in fibromyalgia patients. Other studies have shown significant mitochondrial dysfunction in CFS patients. Both CFS and fibromyalgia patients had significantly increased levels of lipid peroxidation, which indicates oxidative stress-induced damage. Also, peripheral blood mononuclear cells showed decreased levels of CoQ10 from both CFS and fibromyalgia patients.

Another study concludes that deficiencies of various B-vitamins, vitamin C, magnesium, Sodium, Zinc, L-tryptophan, L-carnitine, alpha-lipoic acid, CoQ10, and essential fatty acids may have not a bad thing, as long as it is produced in healthy levels, with the antioxidant-oxidant balance shifted a little to the oxidant side. However, a sufficient antioxidant reserve is needed, and if it cannot be made in the body naturally (due to age or illness), then it must be supplemented.

CoQ10 is a very important antioxidant. In fact, it is arguably one of the two most powerful antioxidants created by your body. The other is alpha-lipoic acid (ALA). Unfortunately, the levels of these two produced by the body fall off with age, and fall off even faster with disease. Fortunately, we are able to supplement them. CoQ10 is important for heart and blood vessels. It is also very important for healthy mitochondria. CoQ10 keeps the oxidants that mitochondria produce from burning (destroying) the mitochondria themselves. Both CoQ10 and ALA make themselves more powerful by recycling other antioxidants, like vitamins A, C, and E. Without ALA or CoQ10, the other antioxidants get only one pass through the body, but if one of these other antioxidants should meet an ALA or CoQ10, then they are redirected back into the bloodstream to work again in neutralizing oxidants. Antioxidants are important to help relieve fatigue because they relieve stress, what is called oxidative stress, in the cells of your body. Then your cells may work more freely and efficiently, so your billions of cells burn less energy to do the same work and ultimately you feel less fatigue. Like stress as you know it, whole-body stress, oxidative stress may also make you feel like "you are running a marathon sitting still."

As indicated, oxidative stress may also damage the mitochondria themselves. So, not only are your cells working harder to do their jobs, they are not receiving sufficient amounts of fuel or energy needed to do their work. This is why fatigue is so closely associated etiological relevance [51]. Other clinical trials have shown the utility of using oral replacement supplements, such as L-carnitine (which increases nitric oxide which leads to more energy), alpha-lipoic acid, CoQ10, and other supplements. One drawback to these studies is that the agents referenced are studied in isolation. Combinations of these agents may have significantly greater effects that they do alone. Clinical experience has been that in many cases, the combination of these supplements significantly reduces the fatigue and other symptoms associated with chronic disease. Long-term use of these combinations often restores mitochondrial function, even for long-term patients with intractable fatigue.

CoQ10 is an important component in the mitochondrial oxidative phosphorylation system. In this regard, it is an important supplement, and individuals with reduced levels, when supplemented, demonstrate increased energy production and reduced fatigue. L-carnitine plays a critical role in mitochondrial processing of ATP. L-carnitine supplementation has been successfully used in clinical disorders that are characterized by low concentrations of L-carnitine. Alpha-lipoic acid as a super-antioxidant is important in mitochondrial function.

Psychosocial stress will also cause fatigue. The stresses of the typical American (western) lifestyle as it affects sleep will effect abnormal changes in hormonal and P&S function that are associated with disrupted or misaligned circadian rhythms, which initiates a cascade of dysfunctions that lead to disease (Figure 2). Sleep dysfunction is exacerbated by aging and accelerates the aging process (Figure 3). Balancing the P&S nervous system, including melatonin function, can restore proper sleep habits and provide restorative sleep (Figure 4). The American lifestyle includes the American diet, with mitochondrial dysfunction. In fact, research has shown that low levels of antioxidants, which may cause mitochondrial dysfunction, lead to fatigue.

There are many things that may also lead to fatigue that may not necessarily cause mitochondrial dysfunction. The stresses of the typical American (Western) lifestyle significantly disrupt normal sleep patterns. This may include frequent jet lag, and people working night shifts, especially if they do not consistently work the night shift[¶]. Two of the most fundamental functions in your body take their cues from daylight: your hormonal system and your P&S nervous systems normally time their functions by the amount and length of daylight as seen through the eyes, including as seen through the eyelids Your body wakes up as your brain receives signals from your eyes, through your eyelids, that day is breaking. The more light you receive in the morning through your eyes, the more energized you will feel. Because these fundamental bodily rhythms are so timed by light, sitting quietly, outdoors, watching a sunrise with your whole body facing the sun and your eyes closed is a great way to start a day that is usually very energized from the start.

While improper amounts of quality sleep will both effect and are effected by mitochondrial dysfunction, poor quality of sleep will cause P&S dysfunction due to circadian misalignment (your day becomes your night and your night becomes your day). Poor-quality sleep includes: too little sleep, too much sleep, and

---

¶ Working the night shift is not the issue. If you work the night shift regularly over a long period of time, seven days a week, with artificial lighting, you are able to train your body to reverse its normal day–night cycle. However, constantly switching from night work to day work, including only on weekends, will lead to sleep disorders.

a diet of convenience; a diet that is characterized by "fresh from the factory" not "factory" fresh. The former is full of preservatives and unnatural chemicals that alter the natural function of the body. By not ripening on the vine and being consumed when available, the body is cheated of the nutrients (including vitamins and minerals) that are only available from fruits and vegetables ripening when and where they are supposed to ripen. Also, by not consuming the fruits and vegetables grown locally, the body is not "inoculated" against allergens (pollen, etc.) that may lead to food allergies, including celiac disease.

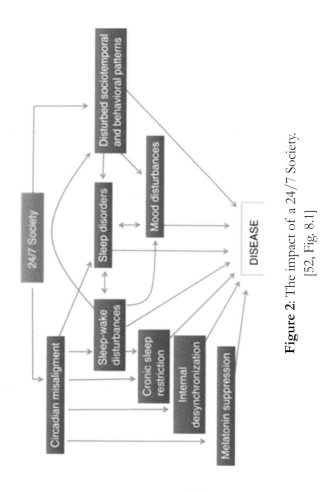

**Figure 2:** The impact of a 24/7 Society.
[52, Fig. 8.1]

constantly disrupted sleep. Too little sleep constantly disrupted initiates a cascade of dysfunctions that lead to persistent stresses in your body, both physiological and psychological, which leads to disease, and if taken to the extreme, will lead to death (Figure 2). Too much sleep also disrupts the circadian rhythm of the body and also causes fatigue. Sleep dysfunction tends to worsen with age and accelerates the aging process (Figure 3). Balancing the P&S nervous system, including melatonin function, can restore proper sleep habits and provide restorative sleep (Figure 4).

The American lifestyle includes the American diet, a diet of convenience; a diet that is characterized by "fresh from the factory" not "farm" fresh. The former is full of unnatural chemicals need to preserve the food, make it look appealing, and simply to make it less expensively. Even most "fresh" fruits and vegetables are not fresh. They were picked too early so they may ship more easily and then artificially (through plant hormones) caused to ripen just before being displayed for the consumer. By not ripening on the vine and being consumed when available, your body is cheated of the nutrients (including vitamins and minerals) that are only available from fruits and vegetables ripening when and where they are supposed to ripen. This is why nothing tastes as good as when it is picked fresh, at the peak of ripeness.

Another issue of the diet of convenience is that the foods that are consumed are not local and not always in season. Many food allergies, including celiac disease, are due to this. Eating local foods (fruits and vegetables) exposes you to the local pollens and such that the plants give off. If you eat some of the plant (fruits and vegetables) every day, your body becomes used to these allergens and you do not react or at least not as strongly. In the case of celiac disease, most

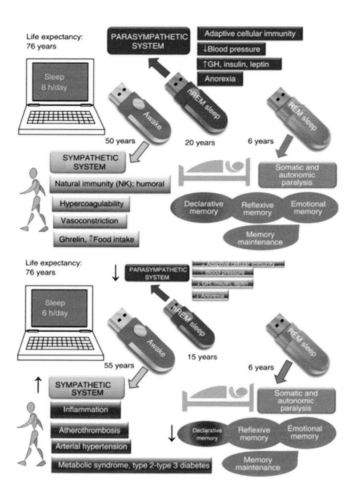

**Figure 3**: Three different wakefulness states (awake, slow-wave or nREM sleep, and REM sleep) must necessarily follow each other for normal health and wellness. (Upper panel) A seventy-six-year-old sleeping eight hours/day will live fifty years in the physiological state or wakefulness, twenty years in nREM sleep, and six years in REM sleep. (Lower panel) A 25 percent reduction in sleep duration over the last forty years of life leads to predominance of the wakefulness state and a reduction in nREM sleep. The effects of this reduction are associated with cardiovascular disease, metabolic syndrome, obesity, and type 2 diabetes. [52, Fig. 8.2]

wheat is grown far from away from you. So if you are sensitive to their pollens, for example, when you eat their pollens, you have an allergic reaction that may range from a "little heartburn" to a full-blown allergic reaction, and regardless of the processing, the pollens are on all parts of the wheat. The opposite is also true. If you suffer from "hay fever," you may do so because you do not consume local pollens. To help relieve this local pollen issue, you may consider taking a teaspoon full of locally grown honey every morning, starting in February. Then, by spring, your allergies will be significantly less severe, if not "cured."

The American diet is also overloaded with chemicals (like preservatives, colorings, and flavorings) and unripened fruits and vegetables and overcooked and overprocessed meats. All of this removes the natural nutrition and (sometimes) artificial nutrients must be returned. Of course the artificial nutrients are not complete, and they often are simply more chemicals that the body is not used to. Often, these chemicals lead to inflammation, which induces oxidative stress, which, when it becomes chronic, also shifts P&S balance and overactivates the immune system, which may lead to fatigue. The point is that the American diet, a diet of convenience, and the stresses of the American lifestyle, even without the psychosocial stresses, help to promote fatigue. The psychosocial stresses merely compound a bad situation. Mass production of foods, which have reduced hunger, may cause allergies and poor nutrition, which typically leads to fatigue.

A sample of what we are talking about is highlighted in the following "day-in-a-life" example. A parent wakes up from a poor night's sleep, prepares for work, drains a cup of coffee, and runs out the door. He or she fights the good fight to get to lunch, which may include a few more cups of coffee to

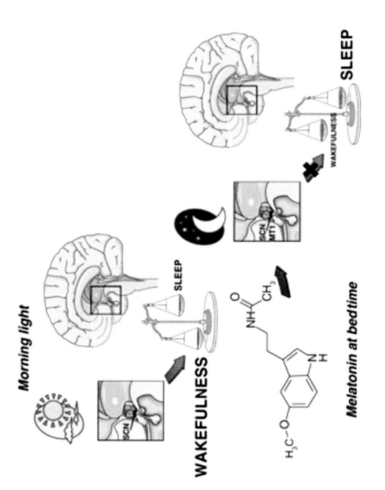

**Figure 4**: Melatonin imbalance with Parasympathetic and Sympathetic (P&S) nervous system (or Autonomic Nervous System, ANS) imbalance, including in the abdominal and thoraco-muscular regions, are known to underlie sleep difficulties and other disorders such as Metabolic Syndrome. The result includes hypertension, increased insulin resistance, and abdominal obesity. [52, Fig. 8.8]

In fact, most foods consumed by people in the US are not grown locally to the consumer. In the case of celiac disease, most wheat that is consumed in the US is grown in the Midwest, or far from the main population centers of the country. This means that stay alert, and maybe someone was kind enough to bring in dough-nuts or the like. Lunch, which is eaten at the desk to save time, consists of prepared food of convenience. He or she fights the good fight to get through the rest of the day, which may again include a few more cups of coffee to continue to stay alert. Then, it is home to the spouse and children. No longer do you cook, there is simply no time, so more fast food so the children may get to their preprogrammed activities. Then the children's homework, showers and bedtime, and perhaps more work from the office, then finally a few hours of sleep before it starts all over again. At the end of the day, you have had little sleep, no nutrition to speak of, no time to laugh and relax with family, let alone friends, and the grind continues. This is too often the definition of success for too many people. All of this stress and the lack nutrients and sleep causes the Sympathetics to be overactive, causing inflammation and oxidative stress, which leads to high blood pressure, an overactive immune system, and excess weight. These may lead to diabetes and heart disease and can cause premature dementia.

An example of the problems with the American diet is that all of the food processing causes vitamin K2 to be processed out of the diet. vitamin K2 is the agent that redirects calcium from soft tissue to hard tissue. The result is that the American population has the highest rate of hardening of the arteries and associated heart disease, and accelerates the onset of osteoporosis. Again, it is fortunate that vitamin K2 may be supplemented. However, that brings up another problem with the American diet. Because there are few nutrients and so much fatigue (which is attributed more to the lifestyle and not the diet, which is a fraud), Americans depend on chemistry to live. It truly is "better living through chemistry." Americans take pills, including chemicals in drinks, to wake up and most people do not breath the pollens from the wheat plant and then consume foreign pollens when they do consume wheat, pollens to which they are not accustomed. The opposite is also true, they do not eat the pollens that they are used to from the air that they breath by eating fruits and vegetables from distant farms. By eating and breathing the same allergens from where they live, people are "inoculated" every day and do not suffer the allergies. An easy way to demonstrate this to your patient is to have them take a teaspoon full of locally grown honey every morning, starting in February. If their allergies are due this lack of inoculation, then by spring, their allergies will be significantly less severe, if not "cured." The point here is that, as you know, chronic allergies and the associated inflammation and poor nutrition from chemical-laden diets, lead to fatigue.

As you know, many medications, poor nutrition (including fast foods, prepared foods, and many of the chemicals consumed), lack of exercise, exercise pushed too far, too little sleep, disrupted sleep, too much sleep, too little relaxation with friends and family (too little, real, laughter), too much work, too much organization, too little spontaneity; essentially all of the hallmarks of the American diet and lifestyle, is a recipe for fatigue. The longer these and other poor habits persist, the greater the possible of dysautonomia. A first symptom of Dysautonomia is orthostatic dysfunction, perhaps the most debilitating symptom. It causes light-headedness when standing and sometimes even when sitting up. Orthostatic dysfunction, in these cases, is when the dysautonomia becomes chronic, leading to chronic and debilitating fatigue, which may not be easy to diagnose, and may be even more difficult to relieve without the additional information available from P&S monitoring.

stay awake. They take pills to eat. Chemistry is now food, rather than food being chemistry. They take pills to relax, including pills in smoke or liquid form. They take pills to sleep, however, few actually get to REM sleep, the deep sleep that everyone needs at least three cycles of per night. They even take pills to make love (have sex). Pills used to be only for the very young and the very old to ensure they had the vitamins and minerals their bodies did not yet, or could no longer, make. With all of these unnatural chemicals and stresses, no wonder Americans spend a large fortune on cosmetics and antiaging gimmicks to not look fatigued and old. (Natural antioxidants do for the long term from the inside what Botox may do for the short term from the outside, for example; and Botox is a poison that, accumulated over time, will also cause fatigue.)

This chemistry-based living is killing America faster than anything else. There is no true (spontaneous) relaxation with family and friends. The time that is spent with family and friends is overscheduled and overplanned and is also Fatiguing. There is little time with children, which causes them stress and leads to anxiety and poor sleep and then fatigue, which in turn causes the adult stress which contributes to fatigue. There is little to no exercise, and that which does happen is often also scheduled and forced, and not relaxed and enjoyable. Many times, the scheduled and forced exercise leaves you more tired and more fatigued, in more pain and may even cause weight gain, contributing to fatigue; and causing you to quit, which contributes more to fatigue. All of this time and money, when exercise should be simple daily activities, like taking stairs, walking to places, gardening, housework, actively engaging with your children, cooking a meal, laughing, etc. Proper exercise is the greatest stress reliever, immune booster, and pain reliever

Early detection of P&S imbalance(s) that define(s) dysautonomia makes it easier to diagnose and treat. For example, many patients do present with both orthostatic dysfunction (an α-adrenergic dysfunction) and vasovagal syncope (a combined cholinergic and β-adrenergic dysfunction). Because it has been difficult to measure both of these simultaneously, at best, most are treated for only one condition and when they seem not to respond, are dismissed as non-compliant. However, treating only one dysfunction typically unmasks the other. Yet both dysfunctions are treatable simultaneously. You may want to start with one and titrate slowly to overcome any sensitivities and improve compliance, but whatever approach you choose, ultimately exercise is the most important therapy; especially for women. Either way, once treated and health is restored, educating your patient in the proper lifestyles and supplements may help them to wellness and a life without persistent fatigue.

While it often takes up to eighteen months or more to normalize severe fatigue patients, this is still considered the "short term." For the long term, supplements are recommended due to the harshness and complicating side effects of pharmaceuticals, which is due to their, typically, off-label use. Again, and to this end, ultimately, exercise is the most important therapy; especially for women. The reason it is especially so for women is that they tend to have physically smaller, thinner-walled hearts than men. It is just the way they are made. As a result, their hearts are more easily deconditioned. Reconditioning their hearts by building them up with exercise increases the stroke volume with each beat. Increased cardiac output improves brain (and cardiac) perfusion, relieving many if not all of the symptoms of fatigue. Due to their light-headedness, reclined or even supine exercises are recommended (some suggestions are included in the known to man. Exercise is certainly better than chemicals. In the case of exercise, stress relief includes oxidative stress, and pain relief is all natural due to the release of endorphins. All of this and more energy to spare, helping to relieve fatigue (assuming you do not overdo the exercise which, as with too much of anything, does harm and may cause fatigue). Again, consult your physician before you start an exercise program, and remember a "low and slow" exercise program (like walking at 2 mph for forty minutes a day) may be just as good, if not better than, a high-impact program, depending on the reason for your fatigue.

In most cases, reclined exercises or even supine exercises are required to begin with because of the light-headedness. With your head low (reclined) or even below your feet (supine), your brain and heart are receiving sufficient blood to support the exercise. In the cases of reclined exercises, rowing; reclined, stationary cycling; and swimming are good examples. Note however, for swimming, using arms and legs at the same time may raise your heart rate too fast (which in many patients' early condition is perceived by the body as a stress), so using only arms for a while and then only legs (with a kickboard) for a while is recommended. The goal is to do this for forty minutes a day, each day, for six months as therapy, and then continue for at least four days a week to maintain. After six months, you are ready to work in other high-impact (stress) exercises (that should have been avoided previously) like weight lifting, running or jogging, contact sports, etc.

In the more severe cases, where you literally cannot lift your head off the pillow without severe light-headedness, the supine exercises are recommended. These start with lying on the floor next to your bed with your bottom against the bed and your feet up on the bed.

"EXERCISE figure below). The graded or reclined exercises may be augmented by the "Modified Dallas Program" to prevent boredom [https://www.dysautonomiainternational.org/pdf/CHOP_ Modified_Dallas_POTS_Exercise_Program.pdf].

### "LOW AND SLOW" EXERCISE
*Supine or Graded (Reclined)*

*Supine Exercises*
*(see Patient Text)*

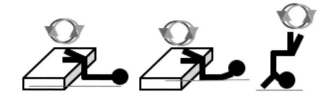

*Graded or Reclined Exercise*

*Seated Rowing    Swimming\*   Recumbent Bike*
*If Parasympathetic Excess (PE): Low & Slow exercise.*
*If no PE, all exercise is healthy*
*EXERCISE IS THE MOST IMPORTANT THERAPY*
*OF ALL FOR LONG-TERM RELIEF*
*\*Swimming: under low-and-slow conditions, only arms or only legs*
*(with a kick-board) to begin with.*

It cannot be stressed enough: some sort of exercise is absolutely required to relieve fatigue—any sort of fatigue. Your patient's heart must be reconditioned—even if they are able to run triathlons. Continued rest only exacerbates their condition. We will revisit exercise again in the "Possible Therapy Options" section.

Then you simply move your lower legs like you were walking at no more than 2 mph; and do this for forty minutes a day (even this, you may need to build up to forty minutes), each day, for six months. During this time, as you improve and just kicking your heels becomes too easy, the next stage is to do as much of the forty minutes as possible with your head raised off the floor. The stage after that is to do your supine exercises using the inverted cycling method with your feet in the air and your head still on the ground (see the "EXERCISE" figure to the left). After this, you may be able to begin reclined exercises as described above. Again, six months or more may be required to normalize your P&S nervous systems and reduce or relieve symptoms. You must remember, your nervous system is like a pendulum. You cannot correct a pendulum with a sledgehammer. It requires numerous gentle nudges over time to correct.

It cannot be stressed enough: some sort of exercise is absolutely required to relieve fatigue—any sort of fatigue. Your heart must be reconditioned—even if you are able to run triathlons. Continued rest, even though you feel that way, only makes your situation worse and possible recovery more and more difficult. We will revisit exercise again in possible therapy options.

There are many causes of fatigue, and the longer these and other poor habits persist, the greater the possibility of dysautonomia. A first symptom of Dysautonomia is orthostatic dysfunction, perhaps the most debilitating of symptoms. It causes light-headedness (dizziness) when standing and sometimes even when sitting up. Orthostatic dysfunction, in these cases, is the cement that anchors persistent fatigue and may make it debilitating, not easy to diagnose, and even more difficult to cure. But that does not have to be you!

# P&S INVOLVEMENT

Fatigue may also be induced by P&S imbalance. P&S imbalance may be induced by mitochondrial dysfunction. P&S imbalance may also contribute to poor brain and coronary perfusion, which often involves fatigue.

## Low Sympathovagal Balance

Resting Parasympathetic Excess (PE) is measured as low Sympathovagal Balance (SB = S/P). A typical patient response is in the figure to the right, above. The whole region that is defined by low SB is in the figure to the right, below. To differentiate resting PE from challenge, or dynamic PE, "resting PE" will always be referred to as "low SB." Low SB is associated with low HR, low BP, depression, fast gut motility (including GERD due to an overactive stomach and diarrhea for the lower GI tract), erectile dysfunction and vaginal dryness, elevated and perhaps excessive immune responses, daytime sleepiness, and, of course, fatigue.

The normal range for SB is 0.4 to 3.0, regardless of the absolute values of your P&S activity. In the Baseline graph to the right, this range covers the space between the two outside diagonal lines. The center diagonal line is "perfect" balance or SB = 1.0. In general, we are born with as healthy a P&S nervous system as we are going to have (the gray area in the Baseline graph). When there is no longer power in either P&S branch, we are at (0,0) on the graph. The slowest "distance" (indicating the longest life) is to stay on or near the center diagonal line. To this end, the normal regions for SB may be refined to include: 1) for younger, healthier patients, the preferred normal range for SB is 1.0 to 3.0 (after all, some younger people need more energy to chase after children); 2) for older, sicker patients, the preferred normal range for SB is 0.4 to 1.0 (as this is the range

# P&S INVOLVEMENT

To understand varied facets of P&S involvement in fatigue, let us return to the "Brakes and Accelerator" analogy.

## Low Sympathovagal Balance

Sympathovagal Balance (SB) is the measure of P&S balance in the body. It is a resting balance, or the balance between your P&S nervous systems measured when you are at rest. SB is one of the most important P&S measures, for this is a basis upon which physicians may titrate therapy in order to "balance" your disease or disorder.

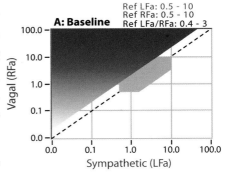

Low SB is too much Parasympathetic activity at rest. As listed in the first paragraph under "Low Sympathovagal Balance" on the physician side, low SB is associated with depression and many other abnormal conditions.

Using the "Brakes and Accelerator" analogy, this is like trying to drive your car with your foot on the brakes. In general, everything is slowed down, including the process of generating energy from the mitochondria. Slower energy production may be exacerbated by poor sleep due to daytime sleepiness. Some think of low SB as your day and night being reversed.

79

that is known to be cardio-protective; in fact, it protects all the organs). Low SB is associated with reduced mitochondrial activity and therefore reduced ATP output. At the same time, it is associated with increased and prolonged immune responses, exacerbating fatigue.

Typically, low SB is a later phase in the progression of autonomic dysfunction. PE in response to challenge or stress often precedes low SB, and low SB is an indication that the responsiveness of the Parasympathetic nervous system has significantly declined, even though it is still over-responsive as compared with the Sympathetic nervous system.

Typically, due to the prevalence of depression associated with low SB, antidepressants are often the therapy of choice. However, the typical dosing of antidepressants causes many side effects that tend to exacerbate the condition. Very low-dose anticholinergic therapy is required. This translates to very, very, low-dose anticholinergic; around one-tenth the dose of the typical antidepressant. For example, where 100 mg daily of Nortriptyline is recommended for depression, 10 mg daily is recommended as an anticholinergic for low SB. Other examples include: 20 mg Duloxetine daily (the lowest dose available), and 0.125 mg daily Hyoscyamine. Occasionally, patients have been mis-prescribed and are found taking the clinical dose of the antidepressant and within two weeks report feeling even worse. Reducing their dosage to the very low-dose anticholinergic level begins to relieve their symptoms.

We find SSRIs have the weakest effect on the P&S nervous systems and often switch patients from high doses of them to the very low-dose anticholinergic listed above.

Because you are sleepy all day, you have difficulty sleeping through the night, and you become more fatigued. As a result, you stop moving, including exercise, and your heart becomes more deconditioned and you become even more fatigued, and the downward spiral continues and expands to other organ systems: digestion, kidneys, reproductive, etc.

The main disorder associated with low SB is depression, and with it, fatigue. However, antidepressants are typically too much to treat low SB. Non-pharmaceutical therapy, as in the Mind-Body Wellness Program, includes the B vitamins, magnesium, antioxidants, and nitric oxide supplements (Nitrates such as beet root powder and

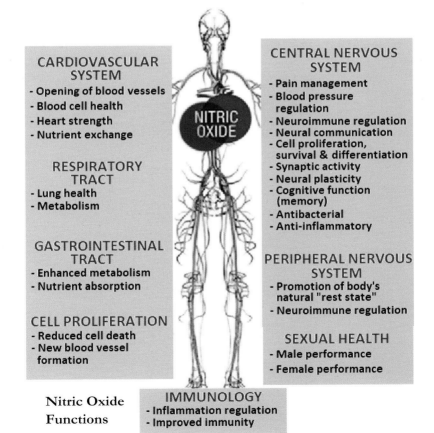

**CARDIOVASCULAR SYSTEM**
- Opening of blood vessels
- Blood cell health
- Heart strength
- Nutrient exchange

**RESPIRATORY TRACT**
- Lung health
- Metabolism

**GASTROINTESTINAL TRACT**
- Enhanced metabolism
- Nutrient absorption

**CELL PROLIFERATION**
- Reduced cell death
- New blood vessel formation

**NITRIC OXIDE**

**CENTRAL NERVOUS SYSTEM**
- Pain management
- Blood pressure regulation
- Neuroimmune regulation
- Neural communication
- Cell proliferation, survival & differentiation
- Synaptic activity
- Neural plasticity
- Cognitive function (memory)
- Antibacterial
- Anti-inflammatory

**PERIPHERAL NERVOUS SYSTEM**
- Promotion of body's natural "rest state"
- Neuroimmune regulation

**SEXUAL HEALTH**
- Male performance
- Female performance

**Nitric Oxide Functions**

**IMMUNOLOGY**
- Inflammation regulation
- Improved immunity

Lastly, pharmaceuticals are typically used to accelerate the relief of the P&S imbalance. In most cases, the pharmaceuticals are short-term (e.g., 9 to 18 months) and are followed up with proper nutraceuticals, supplements, and lifestyle changes that remain, including the supplements at maintenance doses.

## Parasympathetic Excess in Response to Challenge or Stress

Parasympathetic Excess in response to challenge or stress (PE) is differentiated from PE at rest (low SB) by the nomenclature: PE is the abnormal, dynamic Parasympathetic response and low SB is the abnormal, resting Parasympathetic response. PE responses, as depicted in the P&S reporting, are included in the four graphs to the right (on this page and the next). PE in response to stress, including standing up, is associated with the following: difficult-to-control BP, blood glucose, hormone level, or weight;difficult-to-describe pain syndromes (including CRPS); unexplained arrhythmia (palpitations) or seizure; temperature dysregulation (both response to heat or cold and sweat responses); and symptoms of depression or anxiety, fatigue, exercise intolerance, sex dysfunction, sleep or GI disturbance, light-headedness, cognitive dysfunction or "brain fog," or frequent headache or migraine.

PE is also associated with apparent conflicting and confounding responses, such as: anxiety with depression, including as in bipolar disorder; and high BP with depression, including as in PTSD. PE may also underlie Post-Concussion Syndrome and Secondary Concussion Syndrome. The reason for this apparent conflict is that PE is often accompanied by Sympathetic Excess (SE). In all cases, PE should be considered the primary autonomic dysfunction the amino acids: L-arginine, L-citrulline, and L-carnitine). Younger people, under 35 years, typically do not benefit from supplemental L-arginine or L-citrulline, because once the body has enough, it dumps the rest. These amino acids are not stored.

Often, physicians will also prescribe pharmaceutical therapy to help accelerate treatment to balance your P&S nervous systems. However, in most cases the pharmaceuticals are short term (e.g., nine to eighteen months) and are followed up with proper nutraceuticals, supplements, and lifestyle changes that remain, including the supplements at maintenance doses.

All of these recommended therapies are designed to get your "foot off the brakes" to balance your P&S nervous systems.

## Parasympathetic Excess in Response to Challenge or Stress

An example of Parasympathetic Excess (PE) in response to Valsalva challenge, as presented in the P&S monitoring report, is depicted to the right, top.

An example of PE in response to stand (postural change challenge), as presented in the P&S monitoring report, is depicted to the right, below. There are two ways that this form of PE is depicted: 1) the blue portion of the curve in the

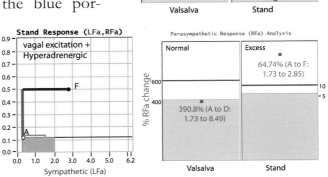

83

and SE secondary. This is due to the fact that the Parasympathetics set the threshold around with the Sympathetics (which are the reactionary branch) respond. Therefore, if the Parasympathetics should increase abnormally, they force the Sympathetics to respond that much greater, abnormally.

PE is common in post-concussion or brain injury patients, and may explain the symptoms that manifest even some time after the injury or event. As you know, the brain's immune system is separate from the body's (due to the blood-brain barrier). In brain trauma cases, PE causes persistent activation of the brain's immune system, even beyond the need for the activation. As a result, the microglia continue to "feed" (be active) and the only tissue left that is not yet mature is the developing and healing tissue. As a result, the brain never fully heals (leading to the "brain fog" and cognitive and memory difficulties). Our experience is that once the PE is relieved, the brain finally heals, and the patient's cognitive abilities return. In the case of some athletes, they get their "step" back even after twenty years post-concussion.

PE is common in PTSD as well as injury in general, trauma in general (mental or physical), surgery, pregnancy (in fact, PE was first discovered in women with more than two pregnancies—we have yet to measure a woman that has had more than two pregnancies that does not have PE, and by pregnancy, we mean through the first trimester at least), major illness or infection, or if the patient had colic as an infant or if the patient has hypermobility or Ehlers-Danlos Syndrome. In all of these cases, there are symptoms of PE (GI upset, depression, sex dysfunction, light-headedness, etc.) as well as symptoms of SE (high BP or HR, anxiety, SOB, palpitations, etc.).

Stand Response Plot, and 2) the right-hand panel of the Parasympathetic Response Analysis plot.

An example of PE in response to both challenges, as presented in the P&S monitoring report, is depicted to the right.

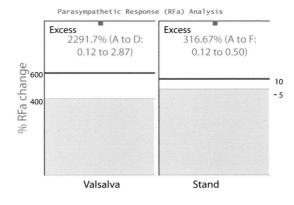

Both the Valsalva challenge (again, modeling your responses to stress, exercise, anger, etc.) and the Stand challenge are both (net) Sympathetic challenges. In all three of these cases, the excessive Parasympathetic responses are causing excessive Sympathetic response as well. Returning again to the car analogy, PE with SE is like trying to drive your car with your foot on the brakes. You may still go, but you must push harder on the gas to get there, causing you to use more gas and over-rev the engine, thereby placing more wear on the engine and brakes. This may cause little touches or stimuli to become "big pain," little worries to become anxieties, or little stresses to become crippling, etc. Ultimately, this additional wear on the brakes will wear out the brakes sooner. The problem is that in your body, we cannot "replace your brakes." Once they are worn (the Parasympathetics), regardless of what the accelerator is able to do, you will still "roll down a hill" and crash. That is your heart attack or stroke in older patients, and in younger patients it leads to CFS, headache, chronic pain, etc. If the accelerator (the Sympathetic nervous system) is still strong, you get to the bottom of the hill faster. . . . Big deal!

PE differentiates vasovagal syncope from neurogenic or cardio-genic syncope as well as from orthostatic dysfunction (including POTS or orthostatic hypotension). In fact, PE may mask ortho-static dysfunction by apparently reversing sympathetic withdrawal (the P&S dysfunction that underlies orthostatic dysfunction, see below), by inflating the Sympathetic response.

Treating PE may take a number of forms: pharmaceutical, nutra-ceutical, or lifestyle modifications. Typically, we work to make the pharmaceutical therapy short term (relatively speaking, since ther-apy may take up to eighteen months; the point is not lifelong).

Pharmaceutically, consider titrating low-dose anticholinergic ther-apy, history dependent, assuming the patient is not also diagnosed with a need for a beta-blocker or anti-hypertensive, or suffering from severe constipation or diagnosed with gastroparesis. However, if the patient is diagnosed with cardiovascular autonomic neurop-athy (CAN, measured as very low Parasympathetic activity at rest), high BP, cardiovascular disease, or a history of beta-blocker, or the patient is a Geriatric, then consider switching to, or titrating, Carvedilol, history dependent, against establishing and maintaining low-normal SB (0.4 < SB < 1.0), as recommended for geriatric patients as cardio-protective. Once titrated properly, the PE will be relieved over time, depending on the duration of the PE. If none of the above: Consider titrating low-dose anticholinergic therapy (very, very low-dose antidepressants, e.g., 10 mg Nortriptyline, QD, dinner, or 20 mg Duloxetine; or anticholinergics for GI or bladder dysfunction, also Hyoscyamine is effective in patients who do not respond to very, very low-dose antidepressants), history dependent, titrated against establishing and maintaining normal SB; this may

PE with SE is a main reason why so many patients cannot find relief or satisfaction from most doctors. They just do not understand that this combination is possible. They have been taught from their beginning that the autonomic nervous system is like a seesaw. They will accept that the "seesaw" may be in balance (normal SB). They will accept that the Sympathetics may be high, causing the Parasympathetics to be low, as in the abnormal resting state of high SB or during normal stress or exercise responses. They will accept that the Parasympathetics may be high, causing the Sympathetics to be low, as in the abnormal resting state of low SB or during normal rest and digest responses. However, the seesaw model

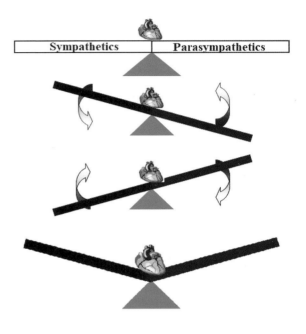

fails beyond that. They have never been introduced to the possibility that the seesaw may be broken and both ends may be high at the same time.

Given that the Sympathetics are the reactionary branch, reacting to stresses (both good and bad) from the level of the Parasympathetics, in all of these cases, the PE is the primary autonomic dysfunction, and should be treated first. Often times, especially in younger patients, normalizing PE (which may take six to nine months or more), normalizes SE (which may take another three months or more), which reduces HR or BP or stress levels (which may take yet another three months or more). The "or more" parts assume that the main also raise resting BP. It is not recommended that the dosage of the anticholinergic be any higher to avoid deleterious side effects.

As discussed above, exercise is the best therapy for long-term relief of fatigue, including with PE. This is the lifestyle modification recommendation. Consider low-and-slow, intensive cardiovascular exercise. Note, with PE, moderate to strenuous exercise has also become a stress for the patient and will only exacerbate PE. This is a six-month program that is designed to "break the bad habit" that everything is a stress and establish a good habit of mild exercise being not a stress. After six months, more strenuous exercises may be added back into the patient's routine. To start with, for the first six weeks, only zero-impact, pure cardiac workouts (e.g., long easy walks at about 2 miles per hour, or very easy bike rides, or walking in a pool with the water level above the belly button) to avoid any tissue breakdown or stress that will stimulate Parasympathetic activity and to avoid (at first) any significant increases in HR or BP that may be interpreted by the nervous system as a stress and exacerbate PE. If the patient is not able to exercise upright or even reclining, they may use the supine exercises noted above.

Although very easy elliptical machine workouts, or swimming, etc., are also zero impact, these modalities tend to elevate HR & BP too fast, causing additional stress in these patients. With these exercises, using only legs or only arms and alternating is recommended. The goal is to only stimulate, gently, Sympathetic activity and retrain the autonomic nervous system to react normally to stresses. This exercise must be for forty minutes per day (you may need to work up to this) for at least six days per week. Remember, a habit has been formed which must now be broken and a new habit formed to disease or disorder is or has also been relieved. The reason for the long lengths of time is because the P&S nervous systems are also like a pendulum. You cannot correct pendulum with a sledge-hammer; you must use many small, "gentle nudges" over time. Otherwise, you will create many side effects or other disorders which might receive additional therapy and create a situation which is much more difficult from which to recover. This is the basis upon which a famous physician (Dr. Sir William Osler; 1849–1918, a cofounder of Johns Hopkins University) taught his students: "The person who takes medicine must recover twice, once from the disease and once from the medicine." Dr. Osler is also credited with teaching the following:

> "One of the first duties of physicians is to educate the masses not to take medicine." (Meaning not to take too much.)

> "The good physician treats the disease. The great physician treats the patient who has the disease."

> "Gentleman, I have a confession to make. Half of what we have taught you is in error, and furthermore, we cannot tell you which half it is." (This is because every patient is different—see the previous quote.)

Relieving PE may be accomplished with one or more of the following (no order of preference):

1. Very low-dose anticholinergics, which are very, very low-dose antidepressants (so low a dose that the side effects—including the suicide risk—are probably negligible). This is used only for the short term until P&S balance is restored, if necessary;

replace it. Target HR or BP is not the goal. For example, after forty minutes of walking, the patient should be able to carry on a normal conversation without being winded. They will still have increased HR and BP and have sweated, but perhaps not within the first fifteen to twenty minutes. The stress indicator is a HR rise that is too rapid. Again, the patient may need to work up to forty minutes to minimize the rise in their HR. Skipping a week starts the six weeks over again. After the six months and a normalization of Parasympathetic activity, activities that might damage tissue or cause more stress (healthy stress) may be returned. In this way, the Parasympathetics are (re-)trained to not overreact to stressful stimuli, making for a more normal

### "LOW AND SLOW" EXERCISE
*Supine or Graded (Reclined)*
*Supine Exercises*
*(see Patient Text)*

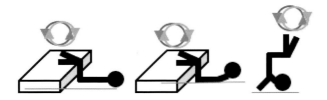

*Graded or Reclined Exercise*

*Seated Rowing  Swimming\*    Recumbent Bike*
*If Parasympathetic Excess (PE): Low & Slow exercise.*
*If no PE, all exercise is healthy*
*EXERCISE IS THE MOST IMPORTANT THERAPY OF ALL*
*FOR LONG-TERM RELIEF*
*\*Swimming: under low-and-slow conditions, only arms or only legs (with a kickboard) to begin with.*

    a. Other anticholinergics may be prescribed that are for GI or bladder dysfunction, also Hyoscyamine is effective in patients who do not respond to very, very low-dose antidepressants;

2. Supplements or nutraceuticals that restore the health of the Parasympathetic nervous system or have anticholinergic effects, the former may include antioxidants, B-vitamins, and magnesium, the latter may include the Hyoscyamine derivative, Phenthonium; or

3. "Low-and-Slow" exercise, like walking at 2 mph or less for forty minutes a day, or as repeated here due to the importance of exercise:

Graded or reclined exercises may be augmented by the "Modified Dallas Program" to prevent boredom [https://www.dysautonomiainternational.org/pdf/CHOP_Modified_Dallas_POTS_Exercise_Program.pdf].

Again, it cannot be stressed enough: some sort of exercise is absolutely required to relieve fatigue—any sort of fatigue, especially if it includes PE. Your heart must be reconditioned—even if you

## EXERCISE BENEFITS

| | | | |
|---|---|---|---|
| REDUCES BODY FAT | WARDS OFF VIRUSES | MAINTAINS MOBILITY | DETOXIFIES BODY |
| INCREASES LIFESPAN | REDUCES DIABETES RISK | IMPROVES MEMORY | DECREASES STRESS |
| OXYGENATES BODY | STRENGTHENS HEART | IMPROVES COORDINATION | BOOSTS IMMUNE SYSTEM |
| STRENGTHENS MUSCLES | CLEARS ARTERIES | STRENGTHENS BONES | LOWERS BLOOD PRESSURE |
| MANAGES CHRONIC PAIN | BOOSTS MOOD | IMPROVES COMPLEXION | REDUCES CANCER RISK |

autonomic response. This program may be augmented by the "Modified Dallas Program" to prevent boredom [https://www.dysautonomiainternational.org/pdf/CHOP_Modified_Dallas_POTS_Exercise_Program.pdf].

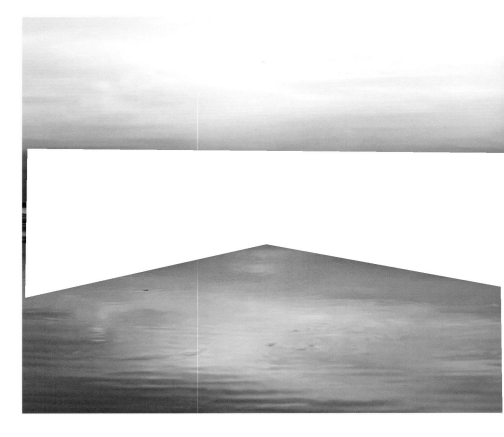

are able to run triathlons. Continued rest only exacerbates your condition. If all you are able to do is lay around all day, then the exercises above that include laying down are even more important. With your feet above your head and moving, you circulate your blood, including delivering more to your brain, and you do a little exercise to work your heart. However, you do not want to raise your heart rate too fast.

See the physician side for more details regarding all three of these therapies.

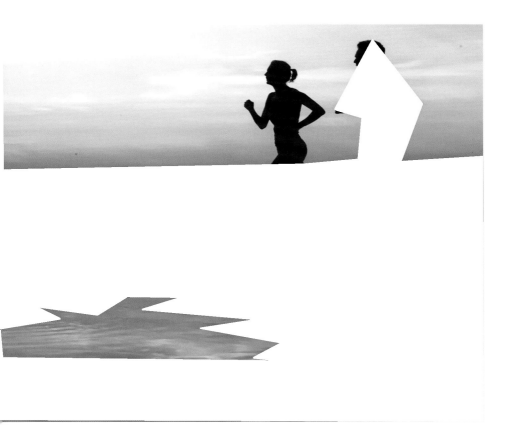

## THE REST OF THESE TWO PAGES ARE FOR . . .

All of the conditions discussed above may cause hypo-perfusion of the brain and of the heart, as well as muscles, and other organs located above the heart, where the heart may be losing the fight against gravity to deliver blood.

Parasympathetic Excess, whether in response to challenge (PE) or at rest (Low SB), both may be associated with other disorders that may lead to fatigue. Note, Low SB is often the latter stage of Parasympathetic dysfunction. PE is the earlier stage of Parasympathetic dysfunction. Think of PE in response to challenge as like being younger and being able to jump—being able to respond more aggressively to stresses. As we age, we may not be able to jump high any more, but we may still be able to walk around—resting responses to stresses.

Parasympathetic dysfunction also effects hormone function, i.e., affecting thyroid and reproductive hormone production, which may lead to fatigue. As a result of these P&S dysfunctions, patients demonstrate subclinical depression and low energy, both are hallmarks of fatigue.

Parasympathetic dysfunction is also associated with sleep dysfunction, another hallmark of fatigue. Sleep dysfunction may involve either non-restorative sleep or difficulty falling asleep or frequent waking during the night. Non-restorative sleep, such as associated with subclinical depression, is typically from resting PE (low SB).

## . . . BOTH PHYSICIANS AND PATIENTS

Difficulty falling asleep or frequent waking during the night,[**] is first associated with PE, then later with Low SB. Either condition is often relieved by low-dose anticholinergic (very low-dose antidepressant[††]). All forms of disordered sleep also lead to fatigue.

---

[**] The reason why people who faint fall down is that once horizontal, the brain and the heart are at the same level, therefore, the brain is fully perfused. If while upright all day long, the brain is only marginally perfused, the brain is not fully awake. Once supine, lying in bed, ready for sleep, the brain is finally fully perfused and is now fully awake. The brain wants to "PLAY!" You and the rest of the body wants to sleep. So you lie there thinking about your day, making lists, etc., but then it is all forgotten as soon as you sit up and the brain is under-perfused again and goes back to sleep. The other possibility (and both may occur together) is that you wake more than twice a night even to go to the bathroom. Again, this is your brain wanting to "PLAY!" It wants to "go for a ride" and gets you out of bed by making you feel like you need to go to the bathroom. Some patients report getting in the bathroom, but not having to go. Again, it is because the brain is now awake.

If sleep disorder is based on subclinical or clinical forms of orthostatic dysfunction, syncope or PE, then assuming a 15° head-down posture for twenty minutes about two hours before bedtime may help to shorten the time it takes to fall asleep. This helps because once fully perfused, the brain is able to wake up, process your day, and prepare for sleep normally, through the normal day-to-night conversion.

[††] Clinical doses of antidepressants, used for anticholinergic purposes, often induce additional (secondary) symptoms associated with too much anticholinergic. Remember, the P&S systems are like a pendulum, they cannot be altered with force, only gentle nudges.

## Sympathetic Withdrawal in Response to Stand

In terms of a tilt-table test, this is associated with neurogenic orthostatic hypotension (NOH) in response to postural change, if BP should decrease by more than 20/10 mmHg. It may also be associated with postural orthostatic tachycardia syndrome (POTS) in response to postural change, if HR should decrease by more than 30 bpm or exceed 120 bpm. As you know, the problem with tilt-tests is that they are not highly effective and, oftentimes, patients do not demonstrate symptoms while on the table. Besides, why do we have to wait for the patients to become so dysfunctional as to have such abnormal changes before we may treat them. P&S monitoring provides additional information to enable a "preclinical" condition (NOH, POTS, orthostatic intolerance, orthostatic dysfunction, or even orthostatic hypertension) to be diagnosed, so that we may treat these patients earlier and relieve their suffering sooner. As it turns out, sympathetic withdrawal (SW) is the common factor in all of these conditions, and therefore they are all treated the same; that is, treat the SW as the primary dysautonomia. By the way, it also happens (typically) to be the first dysautonomia symptom to present, and is arguably the most debilitating.

SW is an abnormal alpha-adrenergic response to postural change. Of course light-headedness is the primary symptom of SW, however, it includes other symptoms which also contribute to the light-headedness; these symptoms typically include:

## Sympathetic Withdrawal in Response to Stand

Again, to repeat the car analogy: if you are at a red light with your foot on the brakes and the light turns green, what is the first thing you do? ... You take your foot off the brakes. Even before you touch the accelerator, you begin to roll, you already begin to accelerate. Taking your foot off the brakes minimizes the amount gas (read that as adrenaline) and acceleration (read that as Sympathetic stress) you need to reach your desired speed. The P&S nervous systems normally act in much the same manner: first, the Parasympathetics decrease to facilitate and minimize the Sympathetic response (read that the amount of adrenaline laying around the body), and then the Sympathetics increase.

Sympathetic withdrawal (SW) occurs when, even after "the foot is off the brakes," the foot is not applied to the accelerator, so blood stays in the feet

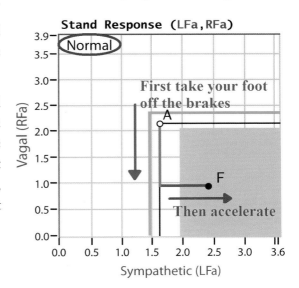

One of the first duties of the physician is to educate
the masses not to take medicine.

—Sir William Osler, Bt

- blood pooling in the extremities, which is often mistaken as Raynaud's disease, due to persistently cold hands and feet.
- poor brain perfusion, which is often characterized by "brain fog," cognitive and memory difficulties, difficulty recalling words, "coat-hanger" pain (in the shoulders and neck), and sleep difficulties,
    - The sleep difficulties are characterized by taking longer than twenty minutes to fall asleep (without medication, including melatonin) or waking more than twice a night, even to go to the bathroom (in fact, many patients report occasionally feeling the need to have to go to the bathroom, but then they do not go). These sleep difficulties are due to the fact that as soon as the patient is supine, the brain becomes properly perfused and begins to function more normally. The patient's brain "wakes up," yet the patient wants to go to sleep. Some even report lying there processing their day, making lists of the things they wanted to do, should have done, or could have done and did not. Their problem is that as soon as they rise in the morning all of those lists are again forgotten because of the lack of proper brain perfusion.
    - "Coat-hanger" pain is due to lack of perfusion of the muscles above the heart, which, like the brain, are also under perfused;
    - Poor brain perfusion may also lead to anxiety, cycled by the "adrenaline storms" the brain issues to demand more blood. These anxiety cycles seem to last at least as long as the adrenaline storms.

and is not helped to the abdomen so that the heart may be helped to send the blood to the brain. (In the Stand Response graphs, 'A' denotes the average resting baseline (seated) state, over five minutes of rest and 'F' denotes the average standing or head-up posture state over five minutes, including the quick postural change.)

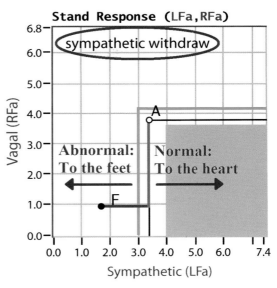

This lack of blood to the brain may account for some or all of the following twenty-five symptoms (see physician side for details):

| Light-headedness | (near-)Fainting | Fatigue |
|---|---|---|
| Brain Fog | Difficulty finding words | Memory Difficulty |
| Pins & Needles in arms or legs | Numbness in Hands or Feet | Coat Hanger Pain (shoulder & neck) |
| Migraine or Headache | Tension Headaches | Frequent Nausea or Vomiting |
| Difficulty standing for long | Chest Pain or Palpitations | Short of Breath (up stairs?) |
| Depression or Anxiety | Sweat too much | Sweat too little |
| Salivate too little (Dry mouth) | Cold Hands or Feet | Dimmed Vision |
| Dimmed Hearing or Ears Ringing | Cold or Hot weather sensitivity | Hypermobility (joints "pop out?") |
| Hypersensitive to light, sound, motion, or touch | | |

- Possible decrease in coronary pressure, measured as a decrease in diastolic BP, which, when paired with the rise in systolic BP due to poor brain perfusion and the associated "adrenaline storms," may also help to induce heart failure should the pulse pressure (the difference between systolic and diastolic BP) exceed 40 mmHg.
  - This is often preceded by fatigue, chest pain or palpitations, shortness of breath (especially when climbing stairs); fainting or near fainting; headache or migraine; hypersensitivity to light, sound, motion or touch, which may also be associated with the possible migraine; "pins and needles" feeling in the extremities; numbness in the hands and feet; persistent nausea or frequent vomiting; difficulty standing for extended periods of time; depression; too little salivation; dry eyes; visual, auditory, or trigeminal disturbances, including tinnitus; and temperature and sweat dis-regulation.

In all, there are twenty-five symptoms or features that may characterize SW, and we base testing on the presentation of four (4) or more. These twenty-five also include hypermobility (including hypermobility due to EDS, which are genetic types) which has no known cure, but is almost always associated with SW and orthostatic dysfunction.

Note, Stand PE is known to mask SW. If a drop in BP from resting baseline ('A') to stand ('F') is documented, then suspect that SW is masked. You may want to prescribe therapy (e.g., very low-dose Midodrine) prn until unmasked.

The diagram below provides a clinically proven algorithm to help detect, diagnose, and treat conditions associated with SW.

## Hypermobility or Ehlers-Danlos Syndrome

You may question why the disorder "hypermobility" (or EDS) is on the list and not other conditions like diabetes. While it is true that diabetes and many other diseases will eventually involve autonomic dysfunction, including SW, hypermobility is a condition that starts in childhood, even if it is not genetic, and brings on severe dysautonomia early. It is a major reason why people (especially females) are good at gymnastics or dance as children (girls), but then seem to crash, typically, as they get into their latter teens or twenties. Because there is no known cure for hypermobility, the best that may be done is to balance the P&S nervous systems to restore quality of life. Fortunately, as far as we know, hypermobility (EDS) is not life threatening. However, because it is lifelong, the autonomics are persistently being pulled out of balance, and maintenance-level therapy will be required lifelong, once recovery therapy has balanced the nervous systems. Further, since hypermobility is lifelong, any other significant clinical event (including pregnancy) often requires a repeat of the recovery therapy. However, once we understand it, we should be able to repeat it sooner.

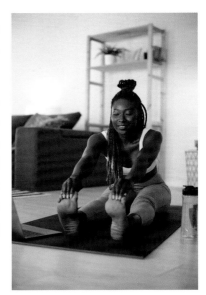

The diagram on the next page provides a clinically proven program to help treat and relieve SW, both in the short term while the dysfunctional nerves are being retrained to do what they are supposed to do and in the long term to keep those nerves doing what they are supposed to do.

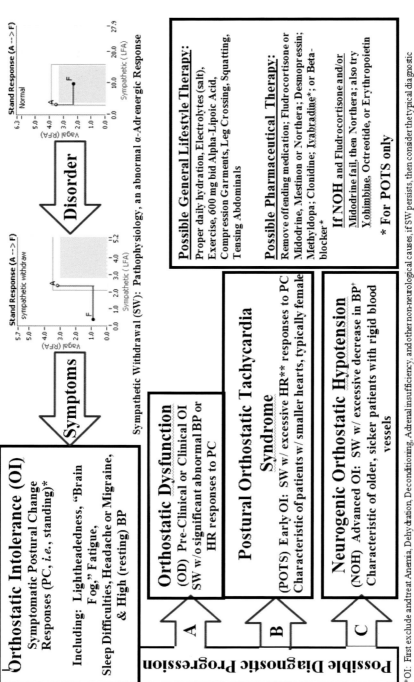

ORTHOSTATIC INTOLERANCE (OI)

Associated with the Autonomic Dysfunction: Sympathetic Withdrawal (SW)

*OI:  First exclude and treat Anemia, Dehydration, Deconditioning, Adrenal insufficiency, and other non-neurological causes, if SW persists, then consider the typical diagnostic progression

** POTS:  Excessive HR response to stand > 30 bpm increase in HR upon standing or an absolute response that exceeds 120 bpm

†NOH:  Excessive BP Response to stand > 20/10 mmHg decrease in BP upon standing

© DePace and Colombo, 2019

# Supplement and Lifestyle Therapy Algorithm for Dysautonomia

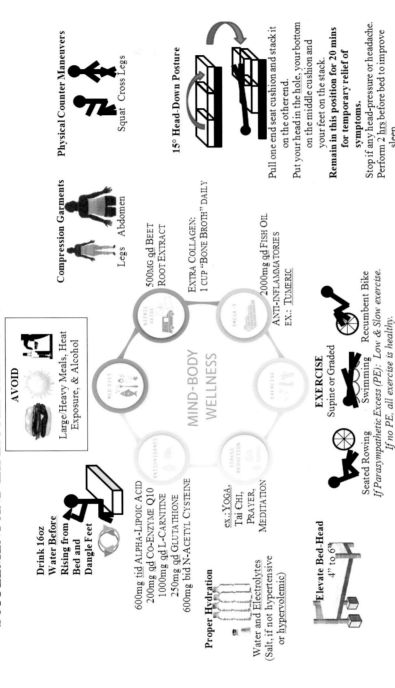

**Physical Counter Maneuvers**

Squat Cross Legs

**Compression Garments**

Legs Abdomen

**15° Head-Down Posture**

Pull one end seat cushion and stack it on the other end.

Put your head in the hole, your bottom on the middle cushion and your feet on the stack.

**Remain in this position for 20 mins for temporary relief of symptoms.**

Stop if any head-pressure or headache. Perform 2 hrs before bed to improve sleep

DO NOT PERFORM WITHIN 2 HRS TO 4 HRS OF TAKING MIDODRINE, DEPENDING ON DOSAGE

**AVOID**

Large/Heavy Meals, Heat Exposure, & Alcohol

**Drink 16oz Water Before Rising from Bed and Dangle Feet**

600mg tid ALPHA-LIPOIC ACID
200mg qd CO-ENZYME Q10
1000mg qd L-CARNITINE
250mg qd GLUTATHIONE
600mg bid N-ACETYL CYSTEINE

500mg qd BEET ROOT EXTRACT

EXTRA COLLAGEN: 1 CUP "BONE BROTH" DAILY

2000mg qd FISH OIL
ANTI-INFLAMMATORIES
EX.: TUMERIC

NITRIC OXIDE

OMEGA 3

MID DIET

MIND-BODY WELLNESS

ANTIOXIDANTS

STRESS REDUCTION

EXERCISE

**EXERCISE**

Supine or Graded

Swimming Recumbent Bike

Seated Rowing

*If Parasympathetic Excess (PE): Low & Slow exercise. If no PE, all exercise is healthy.*

ex.: YOGA, Tai CHI, PRAYER, MEDITATION

**Proper Hydration**

Water and Electrolytes
(Salt, if not hypertensive or hypervolemic)

**Elevate Bed-Head**
4" to 6"

*Proper Exercise and Hydration are most important for long-term relief*

*We understand that this is a lot, but there is a lot going on with you, so let's get started!*

© DePace and Colombo, 2019

Midodrine is the first-line therapy. If Midodrine is not tolerated, then Mestinon is recommended, especially if gastroparesis and constipation is reported. Mestinon is not recommended in cases of persistent or severe diarrhea. If neither Midodrine or Mestinon are not tolerated, then Northera may be considered, especially if reimbursed.

If there is a drop in BP, but no SW, then there may still be orthostatic dysfunction. Possible causes include dysfunctional venous valves, "lazy walls," varicose veins, or blood clots, etc.

## Sympathetic Excess in Response to Stand

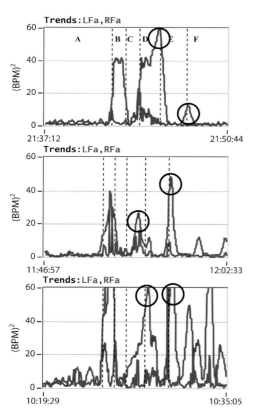

Sympathetic Excess (SE) in response to stand is another source of fatigue. SE is indicated by the Sympathetic response to stand being equivalent to or greater than that for Valsalva. This indicates that standing is a greater stress than the stress of Valsalva. This makes no sense, physiologically. It has been associated with tilt-positive patients. Normally (top graph, left), the Sympathetic response to stand as compared with Valsalva is less than 1:3. Abnormal examples are shown in the bottom two trends plots. The average response is demonstrated in the Stand Response graph to the right (on the Patient side):

All together, including all of the supplements listed above, the thirteen steps will relieve orthostatic dysfunction and the associated fatigue. Pharmaceutical therapy (see the physician side) is often recommended to help accelerate the supplement and lifestyle therapies and shorten recovery, or to help with the busy lifestyles of most of our patients who cannot afford the time needed to invest in their recovery without the pharmaceuticals.

Also on the physician side, we list the reasons why orthostatic dysfunction may occur without SW.

## Sympathetic Excess in Response to Stand

Syncope is another result of the heart not delivering enough blood to the brain, resulting in many of the same symptoms of orthostatic dysfunction. In fact, the form of syncope associated with too much Parasympathetic activity (foot jammed on the brakes while also stomping on the accelerator), known as vaso-vagal syncope, is commonly found with POTS; in approximately one-third of our patients.

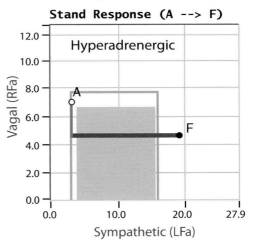

Where orthostatic dysfunction is a result of the lower vasculature not helping the heart deliver enough blood to the brain, syncope is a result of the heart itself not delivering enough blood to the brain. While the end result is the same for both, not enough blood from the heart to the brain causing a

"Hyperadrenergic" (the average is a more than fivefold increase in Sympathetic activity over than for resting baseline). Physiologically, SE represents the "adrenaline storms" issued by the brain to call for more blood and greater brain perfusion. Thereby, SE represents syncope. There are three forms of syncope: vasovagal, neurogenic, and cardiogenic. The first two are able to be positively diagnosed with the more information from P&S monitoring. vasovagal syncope is stand SE (the syncope component) with any form of PE (the Parasympathetic, or Vagal, component) from the P&S test (stand, Valsalva, or rest). Neurogenic syncope is stand SE (the syncope component) without a normal increase in HR from rest to stand (the neurogenic component, indicating that the nerves are not communicating properly with the heart to increase HR appropriately). Cardiogenic syncope is a diagnosis by omission. It is the only option left if stand SE is demonstrated. The P&S test does not test enough of the cardiovascular system to positively diagnose cardiogenic syncope. Combinations are indeed possible, including neurocardiogenic syncope, which is a combination of both cardiogenic and at least one of the other two, the neurogenic component.

Again, SW is an abnormal decrease in $\alpha$-Sympathetic activity with upright postural change, and it is associated with orthostatic dysfunction. While it is not widely accepted, it is possible for this (orthostatic dysfunction, including any of its subtypes) to be comorbid with an abnormal increase in $\beta$-Sympathetic activity while standing, known as ($\beta$) Sympathetic Excess (SE). SE with stand is associated with syncope, which is another condition associated with poor brain perfusion and which leads to fatigue. Because these two conditions are mediated through two different portions of the Sympathetic nervous system, it is possible for them similar set of symptoms, the mechanisms are different, and they need to be treated differently. That is why it is important to differentiate the two. Tilt-table testing is not efficient at this differentiation.

The three forms of syncope are differentiated as follows:

- Vasovagal syncope (VVS) is stand SE (the syncope component, "Hyperadrenergic") with any form of PE ("vagal excitation"). In other words, using the accelerator and brakes analogy, your foot is again jammed on the brakes and you are stomping on the accelerator to no avail, like the fuel line is clogged and no gas is getting to the engine. The therapy, like in other PE situations, is to get your foot off the brakes with low-and-slow exercise or anticholinergic therapy, as discussed and described above.

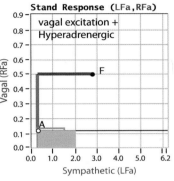

- Neurogenic syncope is stand SE with no increase in HR, like the nerves are not properly communicating with the heart. So while your foot is not on the brakes, the command from the accelerator is not reaching the engine, even if there is enough gas in the tank and the fuel line is clear, there is just no proper call for the gas. This is the hardest form of syncope to treat, and therapy is typically to treat the symptoms, history dependent.

- Cardiogenic syncope is stand SE with normal Parasympathetic and HR responses. This is why additional testing is required to ensure that the heart itself is structurally and electrically sound and that the major vessels leading to and from the heart are clear. Correcting these cardiovascular deficits often relieves cardiogenic syncope.

to be comorbid. This also permits them to be treated simultane-ously (see the SE section below). P&S monitoring, by measur-ing the P&S branches independently and simultaneously, is able to detect and differentiate the two. This is not possible with any other autonomic test because they all only measure total autonomic function and their assumptions and approximations fail to detect, let alone differentiate the two together. The most common form of syncope (stand SE) that is associated with orthostatic dysfunc-tion (stand SW) is vasovagal syncope (Stand SE with PE either in response to challenge or at rest, which is typically a more severe case).

---

*The good physician treats the disease; the great physician treats the patient who has the disease.*

—Sir William Osler, Bt

---

## Autonomically Mediated Arrhythmia

Autonomically mediated arrhythmia, including atrial fibrilla-tion (AFib), ventricular tachycardia (VTach), and bradycardia are arrhythmias that are known to involve P or S dysfunction. A nor-mal instantaneous HR response (upper HR graph, below, top row, left) to the six phases of the P&S test, phases 'A' through 'F' is displayed to the right, and includes: A) resting, initial baseline; B) Paced or Deep Breathing ( you can see the changes in HR due to the six breaths); C) baseline; D) the Valsalva Challenge; E) baseline; and F) stand. An abnormal instantaneous HR response over the

Neurocardiogenic syncope is the most diagnosed form of syncope. Unfortunately, this is not much more than a guess, because there really is not much else it can be, either or both the nerves or the heart. P&S monitoring helps to differentiate Neuro- from Cardiogenic to help specify therapy.

There is one other combination of abnormal stand responses possible: PE ("vagal excitation") with SW. Again, this is like trying to drive a car with your foot on the brakes and not hitting the gas. As with the other stand abnormalities, this combination is also treatable, and both simultaneously. For example, the PE may be treated with low-and-slow exercise and very low-dose anticholinergic therapy, and the

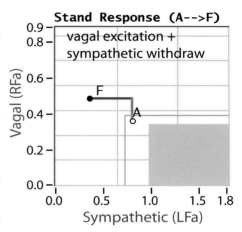

SW may be treated with high-dose alpha-lipoic acid (600 mg, time release, tid), fluids, compression stockings and sometimes pharmacology, including Midodrine or Mestinon; history dependent.

## Autonomically Mediated Arrhythmia

Autonomically mediated arrhythmia, including atrial fibrillation (AFib), ventricular tachycardia (VTach), and bradycardia are arrhythmias that are known to involve P or S dysfunction. These cause the heart to pump inefficiently, leading to poor circulation, including blood flow to the brain. The result may be palpitations or your heart pounding or a feeling of skipped beats, especially with mild exercise, like climbing a flight of stairs. Therapy to establish and maintain P&S balance helps to relieve these conditions. Your doctor may also order cardiovascular tests to rule out heart or blood vessel abnormalities.

same six challenges is displayed as an example (middle HR graph, below, top row, right). In some abnormal cases, the arrhythmia obscures the P&S responses to the challenges, however, the (resting, initial, baseline) SB indicates normal or abnormal. Normal SB indicates that the arrhythmia may not be neurogenic. High SB indicates that the arrhythmia may be Sympathetically medicated. Low SB indicates that the arrhythmia may be Parasympathetically medicated. The other measurements from the test in arrhythmia cases include the BP measures which may provide insight into whether there is possible orthostatic dysfunction. Arrhythmia in response to only some, but not all of the challenges of the test ("Spotty Arrhythmia") also provides insight as to which challenges stimulate the arrhythmia. The Parasympathetics may be implicated if the arrhythmia occurs in only the later resting baseline (section A of the graph), deep breathing (section B of the graph), or (post-exertional) baseline before standing (section E of the graph). The Sympathetics may be implicated if the arrhythmia occurs in only the earlier resting baseline (section A of the graph, suggesting "white coat syndrome"), Valsalva (section D of the graph), or with standing (section F of the graph). Arrhythmia during the baseline after deep breathing (section C of the graph) may also indicate the Sympathetics as a reaction to a strong Parasympathetic challenge. Arrhythmia may cause inefficient blood flow to the brain, leading to poor brain perfusion and therefore fatigue.

## Normal

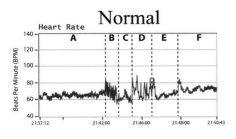

## Abnormal

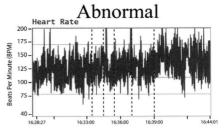

# SPOTTY ARRHYTHMIA

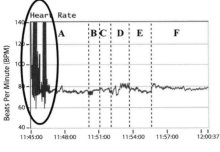

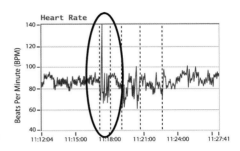

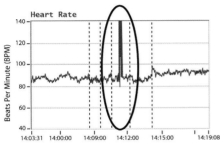

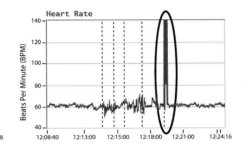

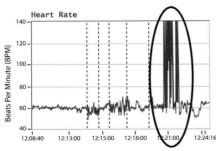

Sample cardiograms (HR plots) demonstrating arrhythmia. The timing of the arrhythmia is a clinical end point. While the arrhythmia inflates the absolute value of the P&S responses, The clinical end point still "tells the story." See text for details.

# THESE TWO PAGES ARE FOR . . .

## Non-Autonomic Causes of Fatigue

Of course there are many other causes of fatigue. Arguably the largest contributors are the American diet and a sedentary lifestyle (in large part due to electronics); some others include:

Non-autonomic causes of POTS, OH, syncope, or Arrhythmia, as mentioned above;

- Poor circulation (e.g., due to Atherosclerosis);
- Low levels of nitric oxide (i.e., due to low levels of nitrates in the diet or low levels of L-Arginine, L-Citrulline, or L-Carnitine);
- Low levels of antioxidants (e.g., alpha-lipoic acid and CoQ10), this may be due to high levels of Oxidative Stress;
- Medications;
- Sleep Disorders;
- GI disturbance and possible Poor Nutrition;
- Psychosocial Stress;
- Psychologically based Depression/Anxiety;
- Lyme Disease, Fibromyalgia, Autoimmune Disorders;
- Mast Cell Disorder;
- Mitochondrial Dysfunction—oxidative stress (perhaps due to psychosocial stress);
- Exercise intolerance;
- Dizziness due to Vestibular (Balance) dysfunction;
- Frequent headache or migraine not from P&S imbalance;
- Collagen Vascular disease;
- Anemia;
- Thyroid disorders;
- Structural Cardiac, Pulmonary and Renal Diseases;

# ... BOTH PHYSICIANS AND PATIENTS

- Malnutrition states, including vitamin and mineral deficiencies
- Chronic infections;
- Cancer; and more.

In most cases, fatigue is a result of deconditioning, not necessarily of (skeletal) muscles, but certainly the heart. We've even said this to people who run marathons. In fact, for "marathoners," exercise is a form of self-medication. They feel better while exercising, but "crash" afterward and may need days to recover from the resulting fatigue.

The heart is also a muscle, a special muscle, but still a muscle and is made stronger with exercise. A deconditioned heart is more prevalent in women due to the fact that they tend to have physically smaller hearts with thinner muscle walls. This is why they suffer from POTS more often than men. The heart has two ways to deliver more blood to the brain: more pressure or more rate. With smaller hearts, there is not the leverage to increase pressure, so the method is for more rate, resulting in POTS. Regardless of the size of the heart, this is why EXERCISE is the only real, long-term curative therapy for fatigue: daily mild to moderate exercise that does not cause too much additional stress, but *must be started under physician supervision.*

While prolonged bed rest may feel like the best thing to do, it is actually the worst. *Prolonged bed rest further deconditions the heart.* If all you may do is lie down, then do so while doing the supine exercises recommended above, slow and easy and as much as possible. Listen to your body. Yes, that little amount is sufficient to get you restarted and on the way to a conditioned heart; and, of course, a proper diet is needed for nutrients and fuel.

# ASSESSMENT, DIAGNOSES, AND POSSIBLE THERAPIES

This is more of a summary and conclusion section, since much of this information was introduced above.

There are many reasons for fatigue, whether chronic or persistent, including: resting and dynamic P&S imbalances, chronic pain (including headache or migraine), chronic illness, poor nutrition, non-restorative sleep, lack of exercise, poor cerebral perfusion, poor oxygen pressures and pulmonary disorders, etc.

## Advanced Autonomic Dysfunction and Neuropathy

P&S Dysfunction may include Advanced Autonomic Dysfunction (AAD), Diabetic Autonomic Neuropathy (DAN), and cardiovascular autonomic neuropathy (CAN). DAN is AAD in patients diagnosed with diabetes, and it is a mid-stage autonomic dysfunction. Typically, earlier stages of autonomic dysfunction are symptom-free, or symptoms are typically associated with other illnesses. AAD and DAN are often marked by orthostatic dysfunction (in adults). However, these early stages of autonomic dysfunction may also be associated with fatigue. Fortunately, there is something that may be done about it at this time, if detected. Therapy, especially pharmaceutical therapy, at this time, may even be short term (not lifelong) and low dose. AAD and DAN indicate high morbidity risk.

CAN is late- or end-stage autonomic dysfunction. It is characterized by very low Parasympathetic activity at rest. In other words, there are no breaks on the car, they have been worn out, and Medicine cannot replace these "brakes." CAN indicates high mortality risk. While CAN may be a normal part of aging, chronic disease,

# HELPFUL HINTS AND CONCEPTS

Again, exercise is arguable the most important therapy for fatigue, especially if the heart is deconditioned. Further bed rest will only exacerbate the situation. Exercise is the most powerful antioxidant,

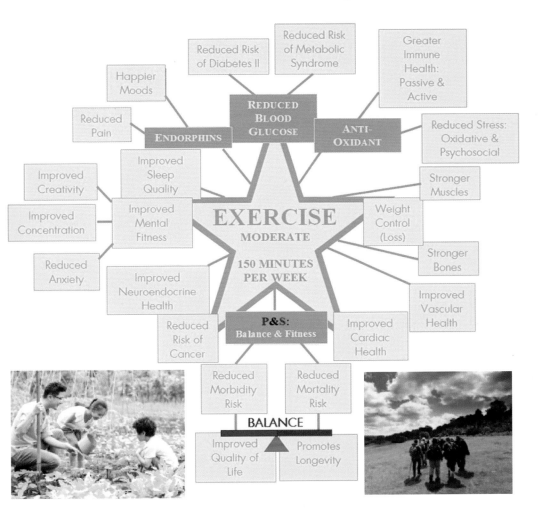

trauma, and poor lifestyles may accelerate its onset. CAN risk is 50 percent greater than in patients without CAN. For patients with CAN with abnormal SB, the risk is even higher. CAN with high SB is considered a better predictor of mortality than low left ventricular ejection fraction.

To treat all autonomic dysfunction or neuropathy, restoring and maintaining P&S balance, both at rest and in response to challenges, is key. This helps to reduce morbidity and mortality, reduce medication load, hospitalization, and re-hospitalization, and thereby reduce healthcare cost for the individual and the nation; all the while, improving patient quality of life and improving patient outcomes.

## Cardiovascular Stress

Cardiovascular Stress is typically the opposite end of the spectrum; it indicates high, resting P or S activity, often associated with growth and development pediatrics, a normal condition, and arrhythmia in adults.

## Parasympathetic Excess

PE (whether Valsalva or stand) is associated with the following: difficult to control BP, blood glucose, hormone level, or weight, difficult to describe pain syndromes (including CRPS), unexplained arrhythmia (palpitations) or seizure, temperature dysregulation (both response to heat or cold and sweat responses), and symptoms of depression or anxiety, fatigue, exercise intolerance, sex dysfunction, sleep or GI disturbance, light-headedness, cognitive dysfunction or "brain fog," or frequent headache or migraine.

PE is common in post-concussion or brain injury patients, and may explain the symptoms that manifest even some time after the injury or event, including fatigue, and immune stress-reliever, pain-reliever, weight reducer, mood-elevator, and much, much more; see figure above.

Low-and-slow exercise is the most recommended therapy for fatigue whether it is due to SW, PE, SE with stand, or abnormal resting states. Whether your "foot is on the brakes" or there is another reason for poor blood flow to the brain or elsewhere in the body, exercise helps to move blood. At first, supine or recumbent exercises are recommended.

Hitting the "brakes" or "riding the brakes" explains the symptoms of fatigue or possible results of poor circulation often associated with fatigue:

- Fatigue: Often patients describe feeling as if they were "running a marathon while sitting still." PE will cause this by causing normal responses to little, normal stresses to be amplified into excessive responses, increasing cardiac function, metabolism, and energy expenditure while doing little if anything.
- "Brain fog" and cognitive and memory difficulties: PE acts to limit the output of the heart under stress. This results in poor brain profusion, which results in reduced brain activity, similar to that associated with depression.
- Sleep Difficulties: If you take more than twenty minutes to fall asleep, or wake more than twice a night (even to go to the bathroom), then your sleep difficulty may be caused by PE. Consider what happens when you faint. Besides gravity working, once flat on the ground, the heart and head are at the same level. Your brain is receiving all the blood it wants; it's happy, you are not, but it's happy. Similarly, after being upright all day (sitting or standing) as soon as you lay down to go to sleep,

weakness. The latter may be due to over-activation of the brain's immune system at the expense of the body's. Treating PE and establishing and maintaining proper SB will help to also treat the concussion.

PE is also common in Ehlers-Danlos Syndrome (EDS) or hyper-mobility. Hypermobility is characterized by "leaky" connective tissue. As a result, things "leak" into the body that should not, causing the immune system to be excessively active, causing the Parasympathetics to be excessively active, and contributing to the fatigue and other symptoms of PE.

## Sympathetic Withdrawal

Any disorder that is associated with orthostatic dysfunction (POTS, orthostatic Hypotension, NOH, orthostatic intolerance, ortho-static hypertension, and their subforms) may all involve SW.

Again, SW is a first sign of more advanced autonomic dysfunction and is another significant contributor to fatigue in hypermobility, diabetes, chronic cardiovascular disease, and neurological and other diseases and disorders associated with orthostatic dysfunction.

Abnormal BP response to stand with normal autonomic responses indicates that the possible orthostasis does not have an autonomic component; consider a vascular study to further diagnose and treat. Recommend proper daily hydration, and also consider titrating lower any diuretic. Orthostasis is a fall risk indicator in geriatric patients and may contribute to elevated, resting BP.

P&S monitoring documents an "Instantaneous" POTS from the Instantaneous HR plot. In these cases, the averaging process aver-ages out the indication ("throws the baby out with the bathwater"), From the Heart Rate plot on the your brain (which has been partially asleep all day) now has all the blood it wants; it wants to play, you want to sleep (you typically lay there processing your day, reviewing lists of things to do and planning for the morrow). By restoring proper brain profusion (blood flow to the brain), your brain will wake up, process your day, and then, with the normal brain changes from day to night, your brain will be ready for sleep when you are.

- For sleep difficulties, twenty minutes of head-down posture, as described, will help you to fall asleep more normally (within twenty minutes) and sleep more restfully through the night. With twenty-minutes of head-down posture, two hours before retiring, your brain will wake up, process your day, and then, with the normal brain changes with evening (from day to night), your brain will be ready for sleep when you are.
  - HEAD-DOWN POSTURE—This is a therapy for SW and associated symptoms, including "brain fog," headache, and fatigue. To minimize pressure on neck, back, hips, and knees, only about 15° head-down posture is recommended. Consider removing an end cushion from a three-seat couch and stacking it on the other end cushion. With your feet on the stack, your bottom on the middle cushion, and your head in the hole from the removed cushion, your feet will be higher than your heart which will be higher than your head. Now gravity will do what your nervous system is not. This may also help relieve evening edema and restless legs. Twenty minutes of this posture helps to restore brain profusion and relieve the aforementioned symptoms. This may be performed any time of the day to help you be alert,

Multi-Parameter Graph Report, the peak HR response(s) to stand is (are) greater than 120bpm. Typically, there is also an upward trend in the HR response after the initial stand response (gravitational reflex). POTS may be confirmed by SW (the causal orthostatic dysfunction). However, POTS may also be accompanied by a form of stand Sympathetic Excess (SE), typically in response to stand PE. Stand SE with PE indicates vasovagal syncope. Stand PE or stand SE (a beta-adrenergic response) masks SW (an alpha-adrenergic response). SW may be confirmed with a concomitant abnormal HR response to stand if POTS or abnormal BP response to stand if OH, as well.

Arrhythmia during stand indicates possible orthostatic dysfunction, and may mask SW. SW may contribute, in part, to increased cardiac workload as indicated by the arrhythmia.

For SW, recommend proper daily hydration (i.e., six to eight glasses of water throughout the day with fewer caffeinated, sugar, and alcohol drinks—sugar substitutes turn to alcohol in the bloodstream), also consider titrating lower any diuretic. If water alone is not sufficient to hydrate (the patient is simply spilling it as fast as s/he drinks it), then add electrolytes. If that is not sufficient, consider very low-dose Desmopressin. If the patient does not tolerate water, consider IV fluids or enemas to hydrate in the more severe cases.

Very low-dose to low-dose Midodrine is the recommended first-line therapy. This may need to be introduced slowly. A little Florinef for a short while may also be needed to help introduce the Midodrine. If Midodrine is not tolerated, consider Mestinon, especially if the patient reports frequent constipation. If neither is tolerated, then the patient qualifies for Northera, and should be pre-certified. In addition to the above, 600mg time-release alpha-lipoic acid, relieve panic attacks and fatigue, and possibly head-aches. If you are diagnosed with SW, do not stay head-down for more than twenty minutes, or the "lazy" nerves in your legs that you are working to retrain with the Midodrine will simply let gravity do their work, go back to being lazy, and prolong your recovery.

- If you are prescribed Midodrine, do not per-form the head-down posture for about four hours after taking the medication.
- If you feel any head pressure or additional headache, stop immediately. You may need to work up to twenty minutes. Your brain is not yet used to all that blood.
- Otherwise, head-down posture may be per-formed anytime to help wake up your brain. For example, a professor who "crashes at 10 a.m. and 2 p.m. every day, put a cot in her office and would prepare for her 11 a.m. and 3 p.m. lectures by laying head-down on the cot. If she was not interrupted by a student, she said she felt like the "'Energizer Bunny' during lecture." However, if she were inter-rupted, she felt like a "zombie."

CAFFEINE is a form of self-medication. The caffeine stimulates the Sympathetics, which helps to increase blood flow, including to the brain, helping to wake and stimulate you. However, caffeine dehydrates and should be minimized in SW cases.

Other stimulants, especially central nervous system stimulants (e.g., Adderall and Ritalin) are prescribed based on symptoms to artifi-cially stimulate the brain. We work to restore proper blood flow to the brain to naturally use oxygen to stimulate the brain and relieve tid has been documented to relieve orthostatic dysfunction, and will help to accelerate the pharmaceutical therapy. Once SW is relieved, 200mg alpha-lipoic acid, tid, is recommended as the maintenance dose. All other therapy for SW may be discontinued.

SW is a fall risk indicator in geriatric patients. SW may contribute, in part, to elevated, resting BP as a compensatory mechanism to prevent light-headedness upon standing. As BP is treated, patients may become light-headed. Reassure them that this is a good sign. It shows that their ANS is being treated. SW with an abnormal BP response to stand is associated with possible (preclinical) ortho-static intolerance; if symptoms, consider therapy, history depen-dent. Treat the light-headedness as needed (e.g., 2.5 mg Midodrine, a vasopressor, QD, Dinner, titrated as needed), history dependent.

Stand abnormalities may contribute to increased cardiac workload which may contribute to cardiomyopathy. Furthermore, SW may lead to poor coronary perfusion and low diastolic BP. As a com-pensatory mechanism, systolic BP may increase in an attempt to return coronary and cerebral perfusion. As systolic BP rises and diastolic BP falls, the pulse pressure increases. If the pulse pressure exceeds 65 mmHg, heart failure may be indicated.

Stand abnormalities may contribute to brain hypo-perfusion, which is associated with fatigue, headache, or depression and anx-iety syndromes. Volume building may relieve these conditions. Approximately 40 percent of our patients are simply dehydrated.

"brain-fog," cognitive and memory difficulties, ADD/ADHD, etc., without the need for artificial stimulants.

STRENUOUS EXERCISE is another form of self-medication. Exercise helps to increase blood flow, including to the brain, helping to wake and stimulate you. Strenuous exercise also releases endorphins which have a narcotic effect on the body and brain and may stimulate the "pleasure centers" of the brain stem. However, in PE patients, strenuous exercise is seen as a stress and the Parasympathetics in these cases will lock away the fat stores and permit only the sugars in the blood to be burned, leading to exercise intolerance and fatigue and possible weight gain.

## CAUTIONS:

If prescribed Midodrine, DO NOT ASSUME A HEAD-DOWN POSTURE WITHIN FOUR HOURS OF MIDODRINE DOSING.

Given that the brain may not, initially, be used to the additional blood flow from head-down posture, you should stop as soon as you feel any head-pressure or headache from the head-down posture. You may have to work up to twenty minutes; that is fine. Remember, additional head-pressure may lead to other undesired symptoms.

With Midodrine, there may be early symptoms, including itchy or "crawling" scalp or goose bumps. These are due to your blood vessels constricting, and you are just not (yet) used to it. Persevere, you'll get used to it. Besides, these symptoms tell us that the medication is working. The same is true for less common symptoms of some heart or chest pressure from the additional blood being moved to the heart.

## Sympathetic Excess

Sympathetic Excess upon stand (SE) represents syncope. Syncope, due to marginally or under perfused brain, may be associated with symptoms of fatigue, headache, depression or anxiety, or sleep disturbance, as well as palpitations or GI upset. There are three forms of syncope: vasovagal, neurogenic, and cardiogenic. The first two are able to be positively diagnosed with the more information from P&S monitoring.

- Vasovagal syncope is stand SE (the syncope component) with any form of PE (the Parasympathetic, or Vagal, component) from the P&S test (stand, Valsalva, or rest). Recommend treating the PE as the primary autonomic dysfunction. PE therapy may be (1) very low-dose anticholinergic (e.g., 10mg QD, dinner, Nortriptyline), or (2) if hypertensive or with cardiovascular diseases, consider switching to or titrating Carvedilol to treat both PE and the (implied) high SB associated with hypertension or cardiovascular disease, or (3) low-and-slow exercise as discussed above.
- Neurogenic syncope is stand SE (the syncope component) with an abnormal (weak) increase in HR from rest to stand (the neurogenic component, indicating that the nerves are not communicating properly with the heart to increase HR appropriately). Recommend proper daily hydration and volume building. Reconsider beta-blocker dosing, if any.
- Cardiogenic syncope is a diagnosis by omission. It is the only option left if stand SE is demonstrated. The P&S test does not test enough of the cardiovascular system to positively diagnose cardiogenic syncope.

HYDRATION: Approximately 40 percent of our patients are simply dehydrated. Hydration is arguably one of the two most important therapies for long-term health and wellness (exercise is the other). Hopefully you will eventually be weaned of the pharmaceuticals, but hydration and exercise (and perhaps some natural supplements) will be strongly recommended for life. This is especially true for all orthostatic dysfunctions (SW) and syncope (SE) patients. Since everyone breathes out a lot of water at night, 8 to 16 ounces of water as soon as you wake up is most important. This should be plain water. If you do not like the taste of water or it makes you nauseous then it is probably the temperature of the water. Remember, your stomach is at a temperature of 98°F, even room temperature water is near 70°F. This is a 28°F difference. This will cause your stomach to contract, shrinking your stomach, making you feel full quickly or pushing gastric juices up into your esophagus and that is what you taste. If any of these are the case, then we recommend sipping hot water to hydrate. Remember, coffee or tea is simply flavored hot water. Skip the coffee or tea (to avoid the caffeine) and just drink the hot water. You should be able to hydrate better.

If you are already drinking plenty of water (48 to 64 ounces per day), consider adding electrolytes to help your body keep the water in your bloodstream. Choose the electrolyte package with your medical history in mind: (1) if you have high BP, then stay away from sodium, tend to more potassium; (2) in general, stay away from sugary drinks, including sugar substitutes; most sugar substitutes turn to alcohol in your blood, which also dehydrates; (3) electrolyte packages have other minerals in them as well, choose ones that will further improve your health; and (4) just as important as the rest is to choose one that you like so you will, actually, drink it.

Combinations are indeed possible, including neurocardiogenic syncope, which is a combination of both cardiogenic and at least one of the other two, the neurogenic component.

A sample Severe fatigue patient P&S monitoring report is presented in the Appendix 2, together with sample instantaneous POTS responses.

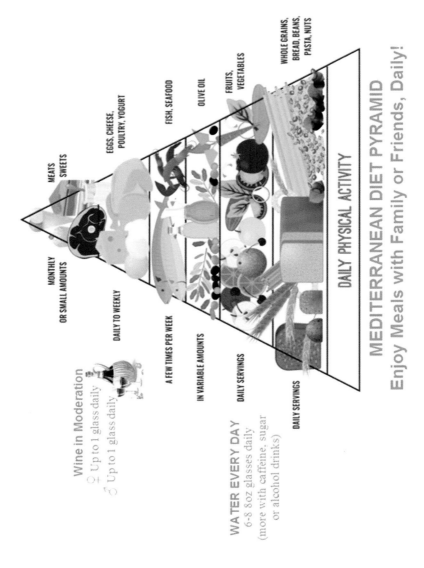

ANTIOXIDANTS (mitochondrial disorder)—a lack of an appropriate antioxidant reserve may cause mitochondrial disorder and thereby cause fatigue. **Alpha-lipoic acid (ALA)** is one of the two super-antioxidants we recommend (the other is CoQ10). ALA is powerful in and of itself, plus it helps to recycle other antioxidants. ALA is selective for

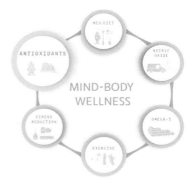

nerves: 600 mg, three times a day, is the therapeutic dose to treat SW; and 200 mg, three times a day, is the maintenance dose after treating SW. It is also the recommended supplemental dose, including for mitochondrial disorder.

**Coenzyme Q10 (CoQ10)** is the other super-antioxidant, and is more selective for the heart and blood vessels: 200 mg a day is the recommended supplemental (therapeutic or maintenance) dose, including for mitochondrial disorder. Other antioxidants include: Glutathione and vitamins A, C & E.

NITRIC OXIDE is an energy producer in several ways: (1) improves blood flow to improve oxygen delivery, (2) improves nerve communications in the brain, (3) Helps to detoxify the body, (4) reduces inflammation, and (5) acts as another antioxidant. It is produced via two different pathways. The primary pathway involves amino acids, which may be supplemented, including: L-arginine, L-citrulline, and L-carnitine. This pathway is rate limited by the amount of L-arginine that can get into the body or is made from L-citrulline or L-carnitine. In younger, healthier people, this pathway is usually saturated. The secondary pathway is via the friendly bacteria in your mouth

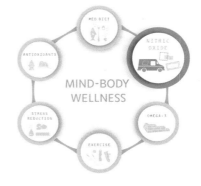

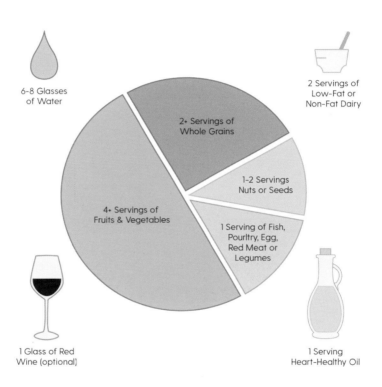

6-8 Glasses
of Water

2 Servings of
Low-Fat or
Non-Fat Dairy

2+ Servings of
Whole Grains

1-2 Servings
Nuts or Seeds

4+ Servings of
Fruits & Vegetables

1 Serving of Fish,
Pourltry, Egg,
Red Meat or
Legumes

1 Glass of Red
Wine (optional)

1 Serving
Heart-Healthy Oil

and stomach. These bacteria are happy to "burp" out as much nitric oxide as you are able to feed them nitrates, like beet root powder. This further supplements nitric oxide in your body, helping to provide the energy you need to overcome fatigue.

DIET—the Mediterranean diet, or perhaps the Japo-Mediterranean diet is what we recommend. A proper diet that is strong on the vegetables, fruits, and whole grains for all of the vitamins and minerals you need for health and wellness, plus healthy sugars and carbohydrates for energy to overcome fatigue; fish and seafood for the omega-3 fatty acids, olive oil and a little red wine for antioxidants and mood improvement, especially when enjoyed with friends or family and laughter, helping to reduce stress.

EXERCISE, as we have discussed several times throughout this book (see the figures on pages 39, 46, and 51), is critical to your health and wellness, including relief of fatigue, both short-term and long-term. Our definition of exercise is an active lifestyle, not necessarily beating yourself up at a gym.

If you are found with Parasympathetic Excess (PE), then low-and-slow exercise is recommended for six months to relief PE, then after, any form of exercise is beneficial. Otherwise, moderate exercise for a minimum of 150 minutes a week is recommended for life. Again, this includes an active lifestyle, for example, taking the stairs and not the elevator, gardening, yoga and stretching exercises, and the like.

STRESS REDUCTION includes both reducing stress at the cellular level by reducing oxidative stress and at the whole-body level by reducing psychosocial stress. The former is relieved by antioxidants, helping to heal the mitochondria, among other things, restoring energy helping to relieve fatigue. For the latter, while stress is a fact of everyday life, we are able to avoid at least some of it. Stress

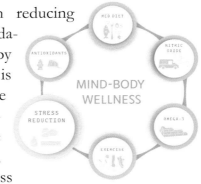

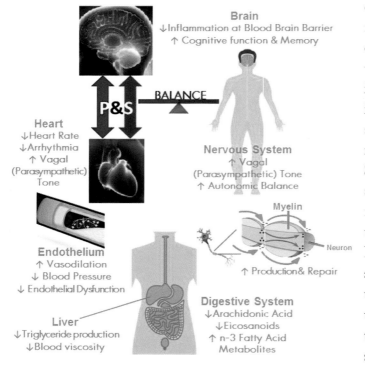

comes in many forms, including: cognitive, emotional, physiological, and behavioral. In general, stress is an abnormally prolonged Sympathetic response. Therefore, most things that will increase Parasympathetic activity will help to reduce Sympathetic activity and therefore reduce stress. The only exception is if PE preexists. See the exercise section above for some treatment options. Reducing stress reduces Sympathetic activity, which reduces, among other things, pain and inflammation, which helps to restore energy and thereby reduce fatigue.

OMEGA-3 FATTY ACIDS are the cellular "building blocks." They are used to repair cell walls and, in humans (and animals in general), help to keep those cell walls more flexible so that they function better, passing in needed, healthy materials and passing out waste materials and materials produced for other cells or functions throughout the body. omega-3 fatty acids, in the form of high-density lipoproteins (HDLs), help to reduce the cholesterol that may become oxidized (e.g., low-density lipoproteins, or LDLs) and form the cholesterol plaques in blood and lymph vessels that clog them, preventing healthy flow. In the correct amount, LDLs

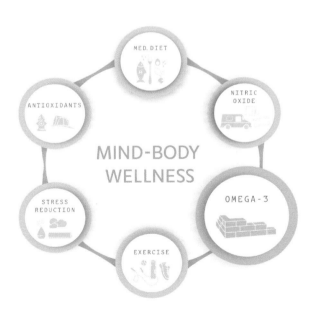

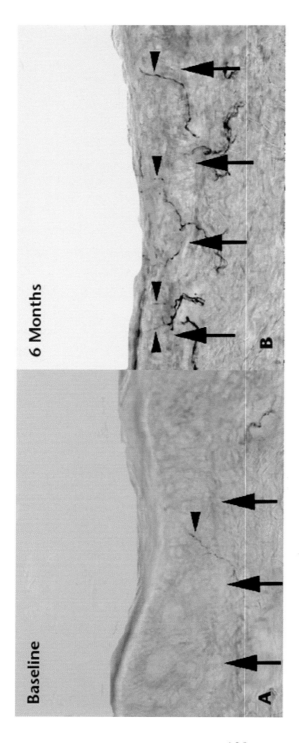

Before and after Methylated Folic Acid therapy from similar areas of skin in the same patient with known small fiber disease. In *the* post-therapy slide you see a proliferation of small fibers, a mean increase of 3.75 nerve fibers/mm. [53]

are healthy and necessary to form structures around nerves that help nerves to function and keep muscles strong. This is why children who are not obese and who exercise regularly should not be denied fatty foods, especially dairy products or the like, because their developing bodies absolutely require all forms of fatty acids, especially for proper brain and hormone development.

SMALL FIBER DISEASE, see figure to the left. There are, in general, three sizes of nerve fibers in your body: 'A-', 'B-', and 'C-' fibers. The first two are primarily sensory and motor nerve fibers. Sensory nerves are those that take signals from the eye, ears, nose, tongue, and other sensory organs, to the brain. These do not include what are called nociception fibers which include pain fibers, as well as temperature-regulation fibers. Motor nerves are those that take signals from the brain to the muscles. These are the larger A- and B-fibers. The C-fibers are the small, typically unmyelinated, nerve fibers which include many of the autonomic nerve fibers and the pain and temperature regulation (aka thermoregulatory) nerve fibers. Dysautonomia or autonomic dysfunction, including autonomic neuropathy, indicates that at least some of the small nerve fibers are inflamed, deficient, or dysfunctional. This is often the beginning of Small Fiber Disease. This also points to the possibility that the pain nerve fibers are also inflamed and possibly dysfunctional. Unfortunately, when pain fibers become dysfunctional, they function all the time, causing pain signals to constantly be sent to the brain. This is the reason for persistent, generalized, whole-body pain, such as that experienced by patients diagnosed with diabetes. Unfortunately, in those and similar cases, pain medication only slows the signals, thereby providing some relief. True, this is important. However, when the pain goes away, the fibers are not healed, they are dead, and lost forever.

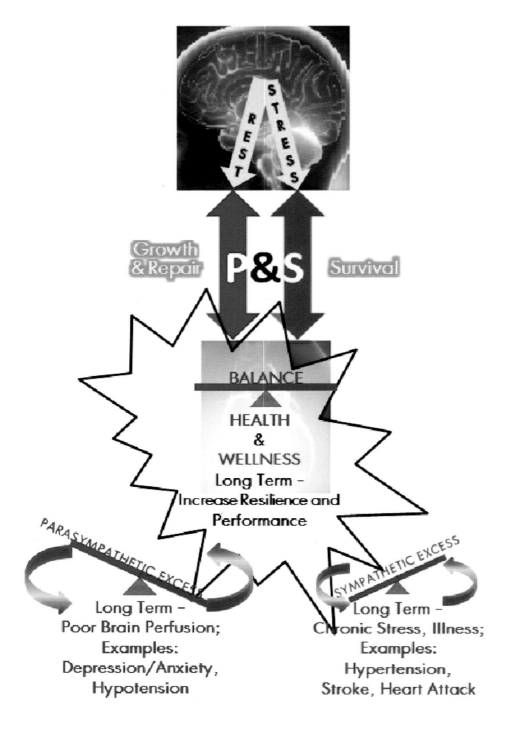

Folic acid (Vitamin B$_9$) is a supplement that helps to heal your small nerve fibers. While over-the-counter vitamin B$_9$ is helpful, especially early in the Small Fiber disease process, or as a preventative, methylated folic acid is the medication of choice. In prescription form, this is Metanx®,[‡‡] which is reimbursed if your doctor orders a Sudo Motor Test[§§] for you and it returns abnormal.

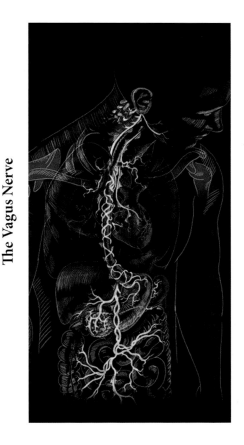

The Vagus Nerve

---

[‡‡] We are not endorsing Mentanx, we cite it because it is the only prescription-grade Methylated Folic Acid available at the time of this writing.

[§§] A Pseudo Motor test is a test of how well your sweat glands are working. Sweat glands are controlled by your autonomic, small fibers.

We, the authors, have developed over time the Mind-Body Wellness cocktail listed below and documented in our medical textbook (DePace NL, Colombo J. *Autonomic and Mitochondrial Dysfunction in Clinical Diseases: Diagnostic, Prevention, and Therapy*. Springer Science + Business Media, New York, NY, 2019.). The medical textbook provides the background for this book on fatigue. The ingredients of our Mind-Body Wellness cocktail are not in any order of importance. All are equally important, especially in the more severe cases. As with any type of therapy, all the ingredients of the Mind-Body Wellness cocktail should be considered patient by patient, based on her/his medical history. Furthermore, patients should consult their physicians before taking any of these agents. This list should not be considered a prescription or a recommendation for anyone.

MIND-BODY WELLNESS COCKTAIL:
- Daily nitrates such as beet root powder, 500 mg/day
- L-Arginine 2,000 mg/day
- L-Citrulline 1,000 mg/day
- L-Carnitine 1,000 mg/day
- Alpha-lipoic acid 200 mg/2x day
- Coenzyme Q10 200 mg/day
- Folic Acid 0.8 mg/day
- Omega 3 1,000-2,000 mg/day

The first four (nitrates and amino acids) are for energy, to boost exercise tolerance and reduce fatigue.

The super-antioxidants (ALA and CoQ10) are to help keep the mitochondria and immune system, and more, healthy and working at peak efficiency. This also helps to reduce fatigue.

Also, nitric oxide and antioxidant compounds are supplements that are known to reduce depression, anxiety, and brain-fog,

ENDOTHELIAL CELL DISORDER—Endothelial cells form a single-cell-thick layer throughout your entire body, separating you from the world around and within you. Think of yourself like a doughnut; your digestive system respiratory system and others are within you but open to the outside world, like the hole of a doughnut. Then, of course there is the outside, like your skin. The endothelial cell layer would be like the glaze on the doughnut, in the hole and all over the rest of the doughnut; this also includes the lining of your blood and lymph vessels. If your endothelium were pieced together and spread out, it would cover an area of more than three football fields. Nitric oxide is a main factor in keeping your endothelium healthy and well. Damaged or unhealthy endothelium prevents the proper exchange of nutrients and healthful elements with waste and unhealthy elements and thereby leads to fatigue. Nitric oxide supplements helps to provide energy through healing of the endothelium. Ankle-Brachial Index testing (ABI testing) helps to document the health of your endothelium.

# Mast Cell

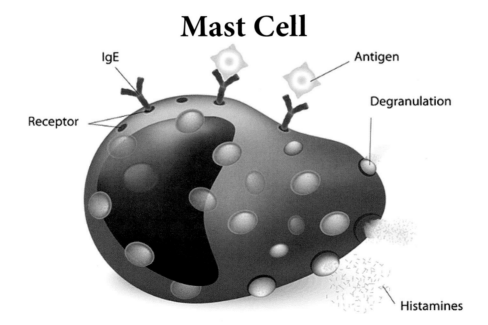

IgE

Antigen

Receptor

Degranulation

Histamines

improve restorative sleep, and more, all helping to reduce fatigue.

Folic Acid helps to reduce pain and the associated lethargy, as well as improve autonomic function, thereby helping to reduce fatigue.

Omega-3 Fatty Acids, among many other functions, help to clear the blood vessels to improve circulation and oxygen delivery to reduce fatigue.

The main modification to this recipe is for cases with SW. In those cases, it is recommended [54] that the alpha-lipoic acid is increased to 600 mg/3x day (perhaps slowly at first and in the time release form to prevent stomach awareness). Then once the SW is relieved, the amount above would be recommended as maintenance dosing.

Fatigue, whether chronic or persistent, involves both low energy and poor coronary and brain perfusion. The above cocktail is targeted at relieving these conditions, with diet and exercise for the long term.

You and your patient must recognize that autonomic therapy is a process that will take some time. The autonomic (or P&S) nervous system(s) is (are) like a pendulum. It cannot be corrected

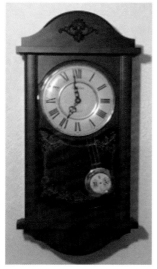

with a sledgehammer. It must be corrected with gentle nudges over time. To that end, therapy will take several months, and perhaps years, to restore your patient's health. Unfortunately, there are no shortcuts to treating Dysautonomia. These are long-term therapies. Pharmaceuticals tend to be recommended during this phase to help accelerate recovery. Again, even the

MAST CELL DISORDER—Mast cells are the part of the immune system and carry granules (storage containers) filled with histamine and heparin. When you are invaded by a foreign or unrecognized substance (i.e., from a bug bite, or a pollen reaction or an allergic reaction, including to food), the mast cells are part of your first line of defense and cause the rashes, hives, or red spots that result. These are supposed to be temporary, short-term reactions while the body identifies the invader and learns how to deal with it. The histamine causes the swelling and local "fever" or "hot spot," and the heparin keeps the blood flowing to the site. Prolonged histaminergic reactions result in what are known as allergic reactions, and in the extreme, may lead to anaphylactic shock. Mast Cell disorder is documented by a twenty-four-hour urine test and treated with antihistamines, or in the extreme, epinephrine (Epi-Pens).

Many medications help to reduce Sympathetic activity (stress responses—"over-revving your engine" in the car analogy) but may induce fatigue if overprescribed, or if you do not actually have excess Sympathetic activity. They are mostly called "Sympatholytics" and include Beta-blockers and anti-hypertensives. There are others that that cause fatigue through sedation. These of course include sedatives and sleep aids, muscle relaxants, opioid pain medications, and seizure or epilepsy medications. Also, antihistamines, some antidepressants, anxiety medications (including benzodiazepines), chemotherapy, some other cancer medications, and medications that control nausea and diarrhea, may all cause fatigue. If you are using a medication and are not sure if it causes fatigue, read the label and warnings to make sure and consult your physician. If you are taking one or more of these, consult your physician to see if your therapy plan may be changed.

pharmaceutical therapies are longer-term than is typical (three to six months for example), and they are always much lower dose, because most are off-label and their side effects are actually additional dysautonomias. Furthermore, many patients have already been previously prescribed high doses of these pharmaceuticals and are often sensitized, and must be desensitized before the lower doses will be effective. Therefore, there are other supplemental and lifestyle modifications that are described above to help in the short term. These short-term treatments may help to temporarily relieve fatigue and one or more of the underlying Dysautonomia(s). Ultimately, we have found that the supplements and lifestyle recommendations of the Mind-Body Wellness Program, or their equivalents, are all required to maintain health, possibly help your patient to Wellness, and to maintain that Wellness for life, including improving your patient's quality of life and possibly providing your patient a longer, happier future. In cases of fatigue, **EXERCISE** may be the only one that stands above the rest, but exercise without the rest is difficult at best.

Studies need to be done with pharmaceutical agents for CFS. Midodrine, which is a primary consideration for orthostatic dysfunction (e.g., orthostatic hypotension and POTS, commonly associated with fatigue) has not been subject to a large randomized trial, although preliminary studies have shown that six out of ten patients with CFS had improvement in subjective or objective symptoms during treatment with Midodrine, suggesting a potential role [55,56]. There is no specific treatment of CFS that has been shown to be universally effective. Some studies suggest that cognitive behavior (psychiatric) therapy may be effective. The very slow rate of exercise therapy has also been shown to be effective in

Ultimately, the most effective therapy, especially for long-term healing and eventually to establish and maintain wellness, is EXERCISE. We cannot overemphasize the importance of *EXERCISE*. It is not a bad word. Just because it is an eight-letter word does not mean that it is twice as bad as a four-letter word! It does not mean you have to go to a gym and beat yourself up. We know you are fatigued. This means you are probably deconditioned, specifically, your heart is deconditioned. Exercise will help to condition your heart, make it stronger, and provide more endurance. This will improve blood flow and circulation to the heart, to the brain, and to the rest of the body. It is amazing what the brain will do with a little bit of blood (read that oxygen). It actually wakes up and gives you more energy. The exercise we recommend for those with fatigue is mild. We call it the "low and slow" program; there are even exercises you do from laying on your back (see above) that is sufficient to start you on your way to an improved quality of life.

All six prongs of the Mind-Body Wellness Program work to relieve and prevent fatigue. The supplements provided in the program are antioxidants, omega-3 fatty acids, and nitrates.

ANTIOXIDANTS such as alpha-lipoic acid (ALA), CoQ10, and vitamins to prevent oxidation of mitochondria improving energy (ATP) production, reduce oxidative stress (stress at the cellular level), and to energize the heart. ALA may burn your stomach. It is now available in a time-release capsule to minimize stomach irritation.

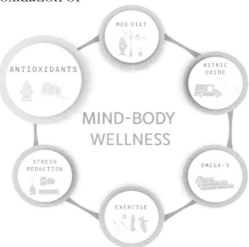

some instances. This is suggestive of the hidden, (dynamic) Parasympathetic Excess (PE) as a potential etiology. No anti-infectious agents have been shown to be universally effective. Medications used in a supportive approach are very important.

There are only two pharmaceuticals (Mestinon and Northera) approved for autonomic dysfunction. All other pharmaceuticals that are recommended for Dysautonomia, in this book and elsewhere, are off-label recommendations. In fact, there are now more supplements and lifestyles recommended in large, multi-center studies for dysautonomia (including dosing; e.g., alpha-lipoic acid, fish oil, CoQ10, exercise, and Mediterranean Diet) than approved pharmaceuticals. In fact, in some cases (i.e., POTS, which is a significant contributor to fatigue, including CFS), exercise is a class IIA therapy.

Having said that, off-label pharmaceuticals can help to accelerate the recovery process that we do recommend. However, let's emphasize the importance of EXERCISE.

Another study concludes that deficiencies of various B vitamins, vitamin C, magnesium, Sodium, Zinc, L-tryptophan, L-carnitine, alpha-lipoic acid, CoQ10, and essential fatty acids may have etiological relevance [57]. Other clinical trials have shown the utility of using oral replacement supplements, such as L-carnitine (which increases nitric oxide, which leads to more energy), alpha-lipoic acid, CoQ10, and other supplements. One drawback to these studies is that the agents referenced are studied in isolation. Combinations of these agents may have significantly greater effects that they do alone. Clinical experience has been that in many cases, the combination of these supplements significantly reduces the fatigue and other symptoms associated with chronic disease.

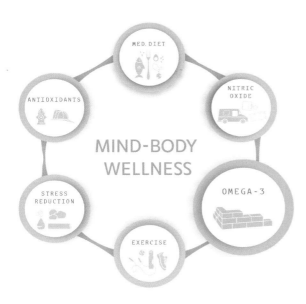

OMEGA-3 FATTY ACIDS establish and maintain a proper HDL-LDL balance to help keep blood flowing properly and to provide the building blocks for repair work (especially brain, nervous system, and heart) mediated by nitric oxide, improving oxygen delivery, removing waste, and reducing inflammation; all-in-all helping to relieve fatigue. omega-3 fatty acids are available from Fish Oil or Krill Oil, and in prescription form as Vascepa®.

Nitrates and essential amino acids are used to generate as much NITRIC OXIDE as possible to energize the body and reduce fatigue. Nitrates are obtained from diet as well as from supplements such as beet root extract. If you do not like beets, beet root extract is now available in (non-prescription) pill form. The essential amino acids that generate nitric oxide are L-arginine, L-carnitine, and L-citrulline.

Long-term use of these combinations often restores mitochondrial function, even for long-term patients with intractable fatigue.

Ultimately, we have found that the supplements and lifestyle recommendations of the Mind-Body Wellness Program, or their equivalents, are *all* required to maintain health, possibly drive the patient further to Wellness, and to maintain that Wellness for life. Together they improve quality of life and reduced morbidity and mortality risk, whether from mitochondrial dysfunction or P&S dysfunction.

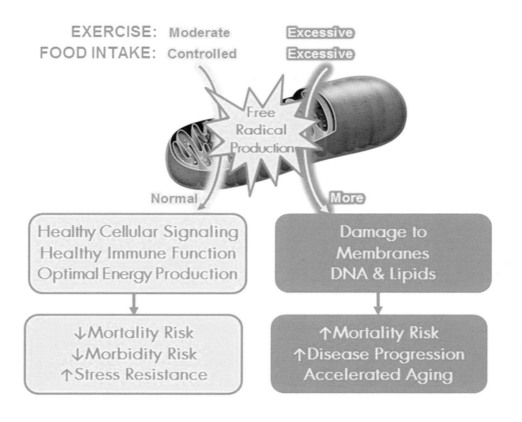

MEDITERRANEAN DIET provides more of all of the supplements, including omega-3s, antioxidants, and nitric oxide. Importantly, it provides these agents in naturally buffered and balanced forms. The Mediterranean diet also provides a platform to help with psychosocial stress reduction through a relaxing meal shared with family and friends.

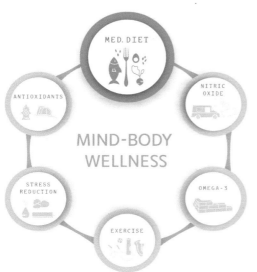

EXERCISE is the most powerful anti-oxidant, plus it circulates blood, improving oxygen delivery and waste removal, releases endorphins which elevate mood and reduce pain, and boosts the immune system. It also helps to reduce stress at both the cellular level (oxidative stress) and at the whole-body level (Psychosocial Stress).

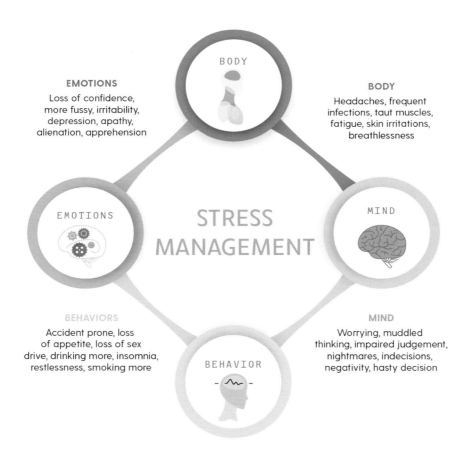

PSYCHOSOCIAL STRESS REDUCTION including medita-

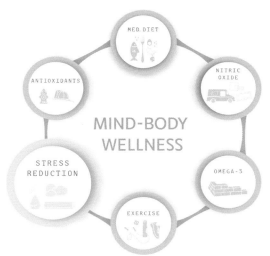

tion, mindfulness, yoga, prayer, time with friends and family, and plenty of laughter. Focus on the positive. Consider everything a learning experience and look for the good and how this stress (a trial) will make you stronger, perhaps not through your own actions but through stronger relationships with others.

Allow yourself to fail, but learn from it. If you do, it is no longer a failure, Learn to laugh at yourself, and laugh with others at the same time. Laughter truly is the best medicine!

The hope is that ultimately you will be weaned of all prescription medications and left with a maintenance dose of the needed supplements. This together with a proper diet, exercise, and stress-reduction program completes your program for a lifetime of health and wellness.

> *The person who takes medicine*
> *must recover twice, once from the disease and once*
> *from the medicine.*
>
> —Sir William Osler, Bt

# APPENDIX 1: THE "ATP PROFILE" TEST

The "ATP profile" test yields five independent numerical factors from three series of measurements, (A), (B), and (C) on blood samples (neutrophils). The three series are:

A. ATP concentration in the neutrophils is measured in the presence of excess magnesium which is needed for ATP reactions. This gives the factor ATP in units of nmol per million cells (or fmol/cell), the measure of how much ATP is present. Then a second measurement is made with just endogenous magnesium present. The ratio of this to the one with excess magnesium is the ATP Ratio. This tells us what fraction of the ATP is available for energy supply.

B. The efficiency of the oxidative phosphorylation process is measured by first inhibiting the ADP to ATP conversion in the laboratory with sodium azide. This chemical inhibits both the mitochondrial protein cytochrome a3 (last step in the ETC) and ATP synthase [50]. ATP should then be rapidly used up and have a low measured concentration. Next, the inhibitor is removed by washing and re-suspending the cells in a buffer solution. The mitochondria should then rapidly replete the ATP from ADP and restore the ATP concentration. The overall result gives Ox Phos, which is the ADP to ATP recycling efficiency that makes more energy available as needed.

C. The TL switches a single binding site between two states. In the first state ADP is recovered from the cytosol for re-conversion to ATP, and in the second state ATP produced in the mitochondria is passed into the cytosol to release its energy. Measurements are made by trapping the mitochondria on an affinity chromatography medium. First the mitochondrial ATP is measured. Next, an ADP-containing buffer is added at a pH that strongly biases the TL toward scavenging ADP for conversion to ATP. After 10 minutes the ATP in the mitochondria is measured. This yields the number TL OUT. This is a measure of the efficiency for transfer of ADP out of the cytosol for reconversion to ATP in the mitochondria. In the next measurement a buffer is added at a pH that strongly biases the TL in the direction to return ATP to the cytosol. After 10 minutes the mitochondria are washed free of the buffer and the ATP remaining in the mitochondria is measured and this gives the number TL IN. This is a measure of the efficiency for the transfer of ATP from the mitochondria into the cytosol where it can release its energy as needed.

# DETAILS

The "ATP profile" tests were developed and carried out at the Biolab Medical Unit, London, UK (www.biolab.co.uk), where one of us (JMH) was Laboratory Director until retirement in 2007. Blood samples in 3-ml heparin tubes were normally received, tested and processed within 72 hours of venepuncture. We briefly describe here the 3 series of measurements, (A), (B) and (C) and how the 5 numerical factors are calculated. (Step-by-step details can be obtained by contacting JMH at acumenlab@hotmail.co.uk).

Neutrophil cells are separated by HistopaqueTM density gradient centrifugation according to Sigma® Procedure No. 1119 (1119. pdf available at www.sigmaaldrich.com). Cell purity is checked using optical microscopy and cell concentration is assessed using an automated cell counter. Quantitative bioluminescent measurement of ATP is made using the Sigma® Adenosine 5'-triphosphate (ATP) Bioluminescent Somatic Cell Assay Kit (FLASC) according to the Sigma® Technical Bulletin No. BSCA-1 (FLASCBUL.pdf). In this method ATP is consumed and light is emitted when firefly luciferase catalyses the oxidation of D-luciferin. The light emitted is proportional to the ATP present, and is measured with a Perkin-Elmer LS 5B Fluorescence Spectrometer equipped with a flow-through micro cell. Sigma® ATP Standard (FLAA.pdf) is used as a control and as an addition-standard for checking recovery. Similar kits are available from other providers, e.g., the ENLITENTM ATP Assay System (Technical Bulletin at www.promega.com), and dedicated instruments are now available, e.g., Modulus Luminescence Modules (see Application Note www.turnerbiosystems.com/doc/ appnotes /PDF/997_9304.pdf).

A. ATP is first measured with excess magnesium added via Sigma® ATP Assay Mix giving result a. This is the first factor, the concentration of ATP in whole cells, ATP = a in units of nmol/106 cells (or fmol/cell). The measurement is repeated with just the endogenous magnesium present by using analogous reagents produced in-house without added magnesium, giving result b in the same units. The ratio, c = b/a, is the second factor, the ATP Ratio.

B. In order to measure the ADP to ATP conversion efficiency via the ox-phos process, the ATP (with excess magnesium) result, a, is used and then the conversion is inhibited in the laboratory with sodium azide for 3 min and result d is obtained (also with excess magnesium). The laboratory inhibitor is then removed by washing with buffered saline and the mitochondria should rapidly replete (again 3 min) the ATP supply from ADP. This gives result e in the same units. The conversion efficiency Ox Phos is f = [(e—d) / (a—d)].

C. In order to measure the effectiveness of the Translocator (TL) in the mitochondrial membrane the cells are ruptured and the mitochondria are trapped onto pellets of an affinity chromatography medium doped with a low concentration of atractyloside. This immobilizes the mitochondria while the other cell components are washed away. The buffers used then free the mitochondria leaving the atractyloside on the solid support that plays no further part in the method. The mitochondrial ATP concentration is measured giving result g in units of pmol/million cells. For the next measurement some pellets are immersed in a buffer (which acts as an artificial cytosol) containing ADP at pH = (5.5 ± 0.2) which biases the TL toward scavenging ADP to be converted to ATP in the mitochondria. After 10 min the ATP is measured again, giving result h in the same units. The factor TL OUT is the fractional increase in ATP:j = [(h—g) / g]. For the next measurement pellets are immersed in a buffer not containing ADP and the TL is biased away from ADP pickup and toward ATP transfer into the artificial cytosol at pH = (8.9 ± 0.2) After 10 min the mitochondrial ATP is again measured giving result k, and the factor TL IN is the fractional decrease: l = [(g—k) / g].

# APPENDIX 2: SAMPLE POTS RESPONSES

Sample instantaneous POTS responses and a severe fatigue patient P&S monitoring report.

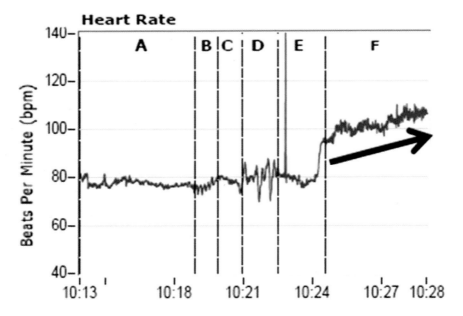

The instantaneous HR response to the six phases of the clinical P&S test of a fatigue patient complaining of all of the symptoms of POTS with SW upon standing (section 'F' of the graph) and a normal BP response, but with a history of a negative tilt-test. The arrow indicates the POTS response.

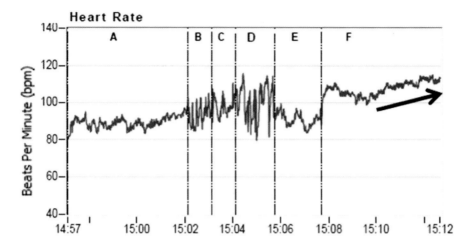

The instantaneous HR response of a fatigue patient complaining of all of the symptoms of POTS with SW upon standing (section 'F' of the graph) and a normal BP response. The spike (at the end of the arrow indicating the instantaneous POTS response) in section 'F' is a motion artifact from the patient sitting down because of severe light-headedness.

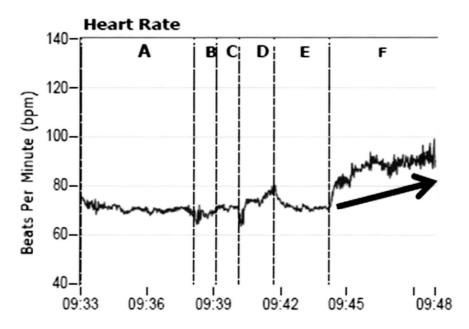

The instantaneous HR response of the patient to the left after three months of alpha-lipoic acid (600mg, tid), Midodrine (2.5mg, tid), and Propranolol (20mg, tid). The HR is reduced the rise in HR (the instantaneous POTS response, see arrow) has begun to reduce and the patient reports beginning to feel better. It took another three months for a significant change in HR to be demonstrated; once the autonomics (SW) are normalized, then the end organ (the heart) will normalize. It took a further three months for the patient to stabilize and be weaned off the Midodrine and Propranolol and weaned down to a maintenance dose of ALA (200mg, tid). Medicated—Propranolol

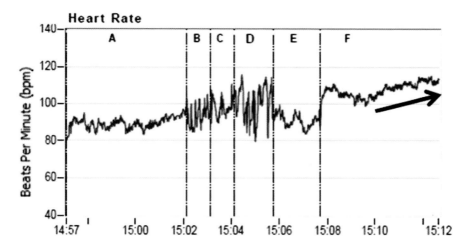

The instantaneous HR response of a fatigue patient complaining of all of the symptoms of POTS with SW upon standing (section 'F' of the graph) and a normal BP response. This patient demonstrates a delayed POTS response (arrow).

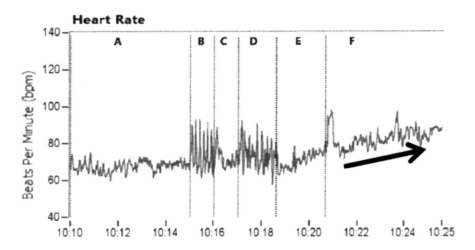

The instantaneous HR response of a fatigue patient complaining of all of the symptoms of POTS with SW upon standing (section 'F' of the graph) and a normal BP response. Unlike the first patient above, this patient demonstrates a normal stand-gravitational response, then an instantaneous POTS response (arrow).

A sample severe fatigue patient's clinical P&S report is presented on the next page. This patient presents with both POTS and vaso-vagal syncope, an occurrence that happens about one-third of the time. As above, the POTS response is demonstrated in the instantaneous HR graph (#1). The orthostatic dysfunction is confirmed by a 16/8 mmHg drop in BP upon standing (#3). The "Stand Response" graph and the "RFa Analysis" graph both present a Parasympathetic Excess (PE) responses to challenge (#2). This is also known as a Vagal excess response ("RFa" is the technical measurement term for Vagal or Parasympathetic activity). In the Trends plot, the peak Sympathetic (red) response is more than one-third that of the Valsalva response (#4), suggesting that is takes a similar amount of Sympathetic activity to stand as it does

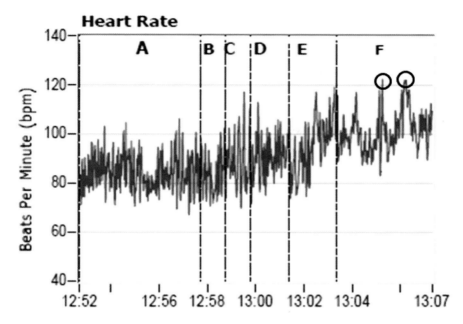

The instantaneous HR response of a fatigue patient complaining of all of the symptoms of POTS with SW upon standing (section 'F' of the graph) and a normal BP response. This patient demonstrates two HR spikes over 120 bpm (circles), indicating pre-POTS, yet enables therapy.

to respond to the very stressful Valsalva maneuver. Physiologically, this makes no sense, and is associated with "instantaneous" syncope, including tilt-positive syncope. Taken together, Vagal Excess (or PE) and syncope indicates vasovagal syncope.

The resting baseline response plot (#5) demonstrates normal P&S responses with a high-normal Sympathovagal Balance (SB). Often with an orthostatic dysfunction (SW, a drop in BP, or an abnormal increase in HR) or with PE, resting BP is elevated or high as a compensatory mechanism to help maintain proper brain and coronary perfusion. High SB will precede high BP. This is an early indication. Low responses to the breathing challenges, in this case a low Sympathetic response to Valsalva (#6), indicate Possible Small Fiber Disease. This may be confirmed with Pseudomotor testing.

# Appendix

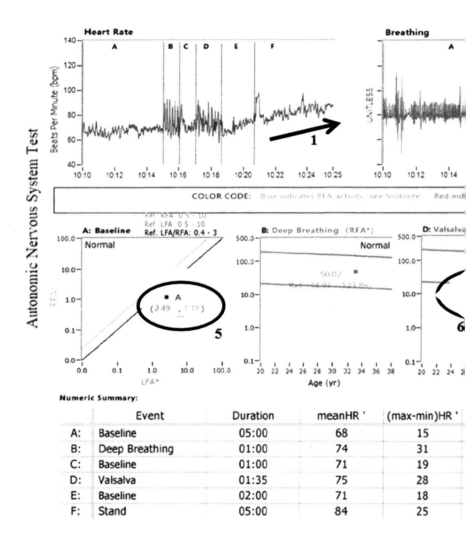

**Numeric Summary:**

| | Event | Duration | meanHR ' | (max-min)HR ' |
|---|---|---|---|---|
| A: | Baseline | 05:00 | 68 | 15 |
| B: | Deep Breathing | 01:00 | 74 | 31 |
| C: | Baseline | 01:00 | 71 | 19 |
| D: | Valsalva | 01:35 | 75 | 28 |
| E: | Baseline | 02:00 | 71 | 18 |
| F: | Stand | 05:00 | 84 | 25 |

A typical Severe fatigue patient: 1) An instantaneous POTS response, showing the persistent rise in HR over the first five minutes after a quick stand; 2) A Parasympathetic Excess response to stand (and short Valsalva maneuvers, both being net Sympathetic challenges); 3) A 16/8 mmHg drop in BP upon standing; 4) An

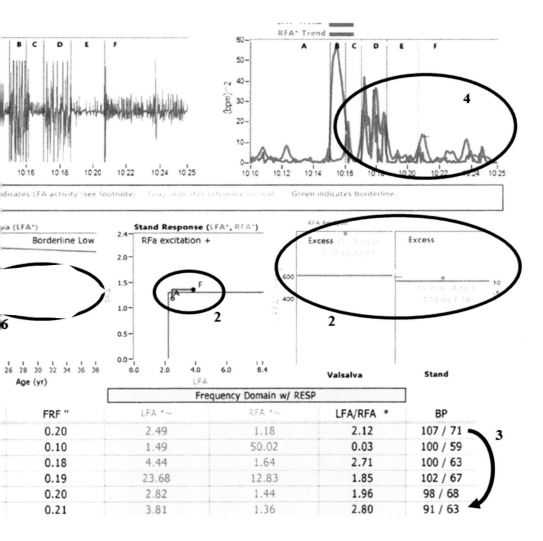

| B | C | D | E | F |

RFA* Trend

| A | B | C | D | E | F | 4 |

dicates LFA activity (see footnote)    Gray indicates reference normal    Green indicates borderline.

va (LFA*)
Borderline Low

6

26 28 30 32 34 36 38
Age (yr)

**Stand Response** (LFA*, RFA*)
RFa excitation +

F
A
6
2

Excess    A to D    Excess

2

Valsalva    Stand

| | Frequency Domain w/ RESP | | | | |
|---|---|---|---|---|---|
| FRF " | LFA *~ | RFA *~ | LFA/RFA * | BP | |
| 0.20 | 2.49 | 1.18 | 2.12 | 107 / 71 | 3 |
| 0.10 | 1.49 | 50.02 | 0.03 | 100 / 59 | |
| 0.18 | 4.44 | 1.64 | 2.71 | 100 / 63 | |
| 0.19 | 23.68 | 12.83 | 1.85 | 102 / 67 | |
| 0.20 | 2.82 | 1.44 | 1.96 | 98 / 68 | |
| 0.21 | 3.81 | 1.36 | 2.80 | 91 / 63 | |

instantaneous (β) Sympathetic Excess response to stand; 5) High-normal Sympathovagal Balance; and 6) weak Sympathetic response to Valsalva challenge indicating possible Small Fiber Disease. See text for details.

# REFERENCES

1. DePace NL and Colombo J. *Clinical Autonomic and Mitochondrial Disorders—Diagnosis, Prevention, and Treatment for Mind-Body Wellness.* Springer Science + Business Media, New York, 2019.

2. Colombo J, Arora RR, DePace NL, Vinik AI. *Clinical Autonomic Dysfunction: Measurement, Indications, Therapies, and Outcomes.* Springer Science + Business Media, New York, 2014.

3. Barnden LR, Kwiatek R, Crouch B, Burnet R, Del Fante P. Autonomic correlations with MRI are abnormal in the brainstem vasomotor centre in Chronic Fatigue Syndrome. *Neuroimage Clin.* 2016 Mar 31;11:530-7. doi: 10.1016/j.nicl.2016.03.017. eCollection 2016.

4. Bested AC, Marshall LM. Review of Myalgic Encephalomyelitis/Chronic Fatigue Syndrome: an evidence-based approach to diagnosis and management by clinicians. *Rev Environ Health.* 2015;30(4):223-49. doi: 10.1515/reveh-2015-0026. Review.

5. Tanaka M, Tajima S, Mizuno K, Ishii A, Konishi Y, Miike T, Watanabe Y. Frontier studies on fatigue, autonomic nerve dysfunction, and sleep-rhythm disorder. *J Physiol Sci.* 2015 Nov;65(6):483-98. doi: 10.1007/s12576-015-0399-y. Epub 2015 Sep 29. Review.

6. Van Cauwenbergh D, Nijs J, Kos D, Van Weijnen L, Struyf F, Meeus M. Malfunctioning of the autonomic nervous system in patients with chronic fatigue syndrome: a systematic literature review. *Eur J Clin Invest.* 2014 May;44(5):516-26. doi: 10.1111/eci.12256.

7. Lewis I, Pairman J, Spickett G, Newton JL. Clinical characteristics of a novel subgroup of chronic fatigue syndrome patients with postural orthostatic tachycardia syndrome. *J Intern Med.* 2013 May;273(5):501-10. doi: 10.1111/joim.12022. Epub 2013 Jan 7.

8. Myhill S, Booth NE, McLaren-Howard J. Targeting mitochondrial dysfunction in the treatment of Myalgic Encephalomyelitis/Chronic Fatigue Syndrome (ME/CFS) - a clinical audit. *Int J Clin Exp Med.* 2013;6(1):1-15. Epub 2012 Nov 20.

9. Booth NE, Myhill S, McLaren-Howard J. Mitochondrial dysfunction and the pathophysiology of Myalgic Encephalomyelitis/Chronic Fatigue Syndrome (ME/CFS). *Int J Clin Exp Med.* 2012;5(3):208-20. Epub 2012 Jun 15.

10. Myhill S, Booth NE, McLaren-Howard J. Chronic fatigue syndrome and mitochondrial dysfunction. *Int J Clin Exp Med.* 2009;2(1):1-16. Epub 2009 Jan 15.

11. Anand, S.K.; Tikoo, S.K. Viruses as modulators of mitochondrial functions. *Adv. Virol.* 2013, 2013, 1–17 doi: 10.1155/2013/738794.

12. Fenouillet E, Vigouroux A, Steinberg JG, Chagvardieff A, Retornaz F, Guieu R, Jammes Y. Association of biomarkers with health-related quality of life and history

of stressors in myalgic encephalomyelitis/chronic fatigue syndrome patients. *J Transl Med.* 2016 Aug 31; 14(1):251. doi: 10.1186/s12967-016-1010-x.

13. Komaroff, A.L. Inflammation correlates with symptoms in chronic fatigue syndrome. *Proc. Natl. Acad.* Sci.USA 2017, 114, 8914–8916 doi: 10.1073/pnas.1712475114.

14. Blomberg J, Gottfries CG, Elfaitouri A, Rizwan M, Rosén, A. Infection elicited autoimmunity and Myalgic encephalomyelitis/chronic fatigue syndrome: An explanatory model. *Front. Immunol.* 2018, 9, 229 doi 10.3389/fimmu.2018.00229.

15. Behan WM, More IA, Behan PO. Mitochondrial abnormalities in the postviral fatigue syndrome. *Acta Neuropathol.* 1991; 83(1): 61-5.

16. Rasa S, Nora-Krukle Z, Henning N, Eliassen E, Shikova E, Harrer T, Scheibenbogen C, Murovska M, and Prusty BK. Chronic viral infections in myalgic encephalomyelitis/chronic fatigue syndrome (ME/CFS). *J Translational Med.* 2018; 16: 268, doi:10.1186/s12967-018-1644-y.

17. Myhill S, Booth NE, McLaren-Howard J. Chronic fatigue syndrome and mitochondrial dysfunction. *Int J Clin Exp Med.* 2009; 2(1): 1–16.

18. Colombo J, Arora RR, DePace NL, Vinik AI. Clinical Autonomic Dysfunction: Measurement, Indications, Therapies, and Outcomes. Springer Science + Business Media, New York, 2014.

19. World Health Association International Statistics Classification Disease and Related Health Problems, 10th revision, ICD-10, 2010, cited 2014, available from http/APPS.WHO.International Classifications, ICD-10, Brown, 2010, G90-G99.

20. Morris G, Maes M. Myalgic encephalomyelitis/chronic fatigue syndrome and encephalomyelitis disseminata/multiple sclerosis show remarkable levels of similarity in phenomenology and neuroimmune characteristics. *BMC Med.* 2013 Sep 17;11:205. doi: 10.1186/1741-7015-11-205. Review.

21. Van Cauwenbergh D, Nijs J, Kos D, Van Weijnen L, Struyf F, Meeus M. Malfunctioning of the autonomic nervous system in patients with chronic fatigue syndrome: a systematic literature review. *Eur J Clin Invest.* 2014 May;44(5):516-26. doi: 10.1111/eci.12256.

22. Agarwal AK, Garg R, Ritch A, Sarkar P. Postural orthostatic tachycardia syndrome. *Postgrad Med J.* 2007 Jul;83(981):478-80. Review.

23. Tobias H, Vinitsky A, Bulgarelli RJ, Ghosh-Dastidar S, Colombo J. Autonomic nervous system monitoring of patients with excess Parasympathetic responses to Sympathetic challenges—clinical observations. *US Neurology.* 2010; 5(2): 62-66.

24. Tomas C, Newton J, Watson S. A review of hypothalamic-pituitary-adrenal axis function in chronic fatigue syndrome. *ISRN Neurosci.* 2013 Sep 30;2013:784520. doi: 10.1155/2013/784520. eCollection 2013.

# References

25. Papadopoulos AS, Cleare AJ. Hypothalamic-pituitary-adrenal axis dysfunction in chronic fatigue syndrome. *Nat Rev Endocrinol.* 2011 Sep 27;8(1):22-32. doi: 10.1038/nrendo.2011.153.

26. Jason L, Sorenson M, Sebally K, Alkazemi D, Lerch A, Porter N, Kubow S. Increased HDAC in association with decreased plasma cortisol in older adults with chronic fatigue syndrome. *Brain Behav Immun.* 2011 Nov;25(8):1544-7. doi: 10.1016/j.bbi.2011.04.007. Epub 2011 Apr 28.

27. Crofford LJ, Young EA, Engleberg NC, Korszun A, Brucksch CB, McClure LA, Brown MB, Demitrack MA. Basal circadian and pulsatile ACTH and cortisol secretion in patients with fibromyalgia and/or chronic fatigue syndrome. *Brain Behav Immun.* 2004 Jul;18(4):314-25.

28. Cairns R, Hotopf M. A systematic review describing the prognosis of chronic fatigue syndrome. *Occup Med* (Lond). 2005 Jan;55(1):20-31.

29. Newton JL, Okonkwo O, Sutcliffe K, Seth A, Shin J, Jones DE. Symptoms of autonomic dysfunction in chronic fatigue syndrome. *QJM.* 2007 Aug;100(8):519-26. Epub 2007 Jul 7.

30. Yancey JR, Thomas SM. Chronic fatigue syndrome: diagnosis and treatment. *Am Fam Physician.* 2012 Oct 15;86(8):741-6.

31. Akselrod S, Gordon S, Ubel FA, Shannon DC, Berger AC, Cohen RJ. "Power spectrum analysis of heart rate fluctuations: a quantitative probe of beat-to-beat cardiovascular control." *Science,* 1981; 213:213-220.

32. Akselrod S, Gordon D, Madwed JB, Snidman NC, Shannon DC, Cohen RJ. Hemodynamic regulation: investigation by spectra analysis. *Am J Physiol* 1985; 249:H867-75.

33. Akselrod S, Eliash S, Oz O, Cohen S. Hemodynamic regulation in SHR: investigation by spectral analysis. *Am J Physiol* 1987; 253:H176-83.

34. Akselrod S: Spectral analysis of fluctuations in cardiovascular parameters: a quantitative tool for the investigation of autonomic control. *Trends Pharmacol Sci* 1988; 9: 6-9.

35. Goldberger JJ, Arora R, Buckley U, Shivkumar K. Autonomic Nervous System Dysfunction: JACC Focus Seminar. *J Am Coll Cardiol.* 2019 Mar 19;73(10):1189-1206. doi: 10.1016/j.jacc.2018.12.064.

36. Bloomfield DM, Kaufman ES, Bigger JT Jr, Fleiss J, Rolnitzky L, Steinman R. Passive head-up tilt and actively standing up produce similar overall changes in autonomic balance. *Am Heart J.* 1997 Aug;134 (2 Pt 1):316-20.

37. Sharpe MC, Archard LC, Banatvala JE, et al. A report—chronic fatigue syndrome: guidelines for research. *J R Soc Med.* 1991;84(2):118–121.

38. Fukuda K, Straus SE, Hickie I, Sharpe MC, Dobbins JG, Komaroff A; International Chronic Fatigue Syndrome Study Group. The chronic fatigue

syndrome: a comprehensive approach to its definition and study. *Ann Intern Med.* 1994;121(12):953–959.

39. National Collaborating Centre for Primary Care (Great Britain), Royal College of General Practitioners. Chronic Fatigue Syndrome/Myalgic Encephalomyelitis (or Encephalopathy): Diagnosis and Management of Chronic Fatigue Syndrome/ Myalgic Encephalomyelitis (or Encephalopathy) in Adults and Children. London, England: National Collaborating Centre for Primary Care, Royal College of General Practitioners; 2007.

40. Costigan A, Elliott C, McDonald C, Newton JL. Orthostatic symptoms predict functional capacity in chronic fatigue syndrome: implications for management. *QJM.* 2010 Aug;103(8):589-95. doi: 10.1093/qjmed/hcq094. Epub 2010 Jun 9.

41. Wolther HH, Bogaard HJ, de Vries PM. The technique of impedance cardiography. *Eur Heart J.* 1997 Sep;18(9):1396-403.

42. Jones DE, Gray J, Frith J, Newton JL. Fatigue severity remains stable over time and independently associated with orthostatic symptoms in chronic fatigue syndrome: a longitudinal study. *J Intern Med.* 2011 Feb;269(2):182-8. doi: 10.1111/j.1365-2796.2010.02306.x. Epub 2010 Nov 14.

43. Hollingsworth KG, Jones DE, Taylor R, Blamire AM, Newton JL. Impaired cardiovascular response to standing in chronic fatigue syndrome. *Eur J Clin Invest.* 2010 Jul;40(7):608-15. doi: 10.1111/j.1365-2362.2010.02310.x. Epub 2010 May 23. PMID: 20497461.

44. Okamoto LE, Raj SR, Peltier A, Gamboa A, Shibao C, Diedrich A, Black BK, Robertson D, Biaggioni I. Neurohumoral and haemodynamic profile in postural tachycardia and chronic fatigue syndromes. *Clin Sci* (Lond). 2012 Feb;122(4):183-92. doi: 10.1042/CS20110200. PMID: 21906029.

45. Filler K, Lyon D, Bennett J, McCain N, Elswick R, Lukkahatai N, Saligan LN. Association of Mitochondrial Dysfunction and Fatigue: A Review of the Literature. *BBA Clin.* 2014 Jun 1;1:12-23.

46. Singh B, Singh R. Mitochondrial dysfunction and chronic fatigue syndromes: Issues in clinical care. *IOSR-JDMS.* 2014; 13(5): 30-3 e-ISSN: 2279-0853, p-ISSN: 2279-0861.

47. Sack MN, Fyhrquist FY, Saijonmaa OJ, Fuster V, Kovacic JC. Basic Biology of Oxidative Stress and the Cardiovascular System: Part 1 of a 3-Part Series. *J Am Coll Cardiol.* 2017 Jul 11;70(2):196-211. doi: 10.1016/j.jacc.2017.05.034.

48. Adly AAM. Oxidative Stress and Disease: An Updated Review. *Research Journal of Immunology.* 2010; 3: 129-145.

49. Seung-Kwon Myung, Woong Ju, Belong Cho, Seung-Won Oh, Sang Min Park, Bon-Kwon Koo, Byung-Joo Park. Efficacy of vitamin and antioxidant supplements in prevention of cardiovascular disease: systematic review and meta-analysis of

# References

randomised controlled trials  *BMJ*. 2013; 346: f10. Published online 2013 Jan 18. doi: 10.1136/bmj.f10

50.  Castro-Marrero J, Cordero MD, Sáez-Francas N, Jimenez-Gutierrez C, Aguilar-Montilla FJ, Aliste L, Alegre-Martin J.  Could mitochondrial dysfunction be a differentiating marker between chronic fatigue syndrome and fibromyalgia?  *Antioxid Redox Signal*. 2013 Nov 20;19(15):1855-60. doi: 10.1089/ars.2013.5346. Epub 2013 May 29.

51.  Singh B, Singh R.  Mitochondrial dysfunction and chronic fatigue syndromes: Issues in clinical care.  *IOSR-JDMS*.  2014; 13(5): 30-3  e-ISSN: 2279-0853, p-ISSN: 2279-0861.

52.  Cardinali DP.  Autonomic Nervous System: *Basic and Clinical Aspects*.  Springer International Publishing AG, 2018.

53.  Jacobs AM, Dunlei C.  Management of diabetic small-fiber neuropathy with combination L-methylfolate, methylcobalamin, and pyridoxal 5'-phosphate. *Rev Neurolog Dis*. 2011; 8 1-2: 39-47.

54.  Murray GL, Colombo J.  (R)alpha lipoic acid is a safe, effective pharmacologic therapy of chronic orthostatic hypotension associated with low sympathetic tone. 2020; *Clin Cardiol Cardiovasc Med*. 4: 6-12..

55.  Naschitz J, Dreyfuss D, Yeshurun D, Rosner I.  Midodrine treatment for chronic fatigue syndrome.  *Postgrad Med J*. 2004 Apr;80(942):230-2.

56.  Naschitz JE, Rosner I, Rozenbaum M, Naschitz S, Musafia-Priselac R, Shaviv N, Fields M, Isseroff H, Zuckerman E, Yeshurun D, Sabo E.  The head-up tilt test with haemodynamic instability score in diagnosing chronic fatigue syndrome.  *QJM*. 2003 Feb;96(2):133-42.

57.  Singh B, Singh R.  Mitochondrial dysfunction and chronic fatigue syndromes: Issues in clinical care.  *IOSR-JDMS*.  2014; 13(5): 30-3  e-ISSN: 2279-0853, p-ISSN: 2279-0861.